THE HOTBED COLLECTIVE

The Hotbed Collective is a collection of women –
with writers Lisa Williams and Anniki Sommer-
ville at the forefront – whose mission is to make
life better, one orgasm at a time. They believe
that sex, relationships and body confidence are
feminist issues which shouldn't be ignored.
Their podcast *The Hotbed* has given a platform
to doctors, therapists, bloggers, politicians and
celebrities to talk honestly about female pleasure
in all its forms.

THE HOTBED COLLECTIVE

More Orgasms Please

Why Female Pleasure Matters

VINTAGE

1 3 5 7 9 10 8 6 4 2

Vintage
20 Vauxhall Bridge Road,
London SW1V 2SA

Vintage is part of the Penguin Random House group of companies
whose addresses can be found at global.penguinrandomhouse.com

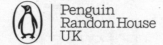

Penguin
Random House
UK

First published by Vintage in 2020
First published in the UK by Square Peg in 2019

penguin.co.uk/vintage

A CIP catalogue record for this book is available from the
British Library

ISBN 9781529110852

Printed and bound in Great Britain by Clays Ltd, Elcograf S.p.A.

Penguin Random House is committed to a sustainable future
for our business, our readers and our planet. This book is
made from Forest Stewardship Council® certified paper.

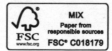

FOR NANCY FRIDAY

CONTENTS

FOREWORD

by Cherry Healey, founding Hotbed Collective member

For me, Hotbed was born out of embarrassment and confusion: embarrassment that, at thirty, I had to admit to myself that, after years of pretending that I was nonplussed, I really enjoyed sex. I was really interested in sex. And I was also confused about the mixed messages about sex: that women shouldn't admit to enjoying sex or, if they don't enjoy it, take steps to learn how they could. And that, in the bedroom, they should always act as if they really enjoy sex, and that there's only one type of sex they should enjoy. I was confused at the message that fun, hot sex had to be over once a relationship tipped over the 'several years' mark, and that you absolutely definitely had to accept the Death Of Sex after kids.

But I was also confused by the excitement and fun of the conversations that I was having with female friends: I was clearly not the only one who was curious. But it was almost clandestine, and we acknowledged, without verbalising, that it was a bit naughty to be a woman and be openly sexual. Society, even our apparently liberal one, had told us again and again that a woman who loves sex is not to be trusted and certainly not someone you want as a wife (insert awful terms like slag etc. etc. that I can't bring myself to write).

And yet there's nothing wrong with me or my friends: we get our kids to school on time, we brush their hair — and sometimes our own — we pay our bills on time, write killer proposals at work, are often the only ones to remember Jeff's birthday, help our elderly neighbours, and yet also want hot, hot sex.

And the more I searched, the more I realised that there were almost no women I related to talking with confidence about hot, hot sex in a public forum. I wondered, do I need to go to an S&M basement in order to talk with confidence about sex?

And then I met Anniki and Lisa — and Hotbed was born. We are all different in what we like and want from sex but what we all absolutely agree on is that there is a huge lack of conversation and a huge amount of shame around female pleasure.

The Hotbed Collective started as a website with articles written by us and anyone who wanted to contribute (turns out, a lot) and then it turned into live events, then a podcast and now it is a book. We have always had the intention of giving women the confidence to talk openly and freely about sex — with absolutely no shame and hopefully some joy. This book outlines how women have been kept ignorant about their sexuality or made to feel ashamed of it (to the point where many women won't even go to the doctor when they're worried about something, for fear of saying the words vulva or vagina out loud), and how damaging that is to their confidence and relationships. It also offers ideas and advice on how to change that.

Sex chat doesn't have to be salacious and seedy or boring and medical. We need to reclaim sex as a normal, healthy, fun, exciting part of life. There are a thousand types of gym classes and gym outfits and health drinks and health powders and dumbbells and kettlebells and eight hundred different workout videos online and yet sex, which can be just as important to your health and the health of your relationship, is not often talked about outside of medical textbooks, unrealistic how-to manuals and, very sadly, court cases. I dare you to talk to your friends, or your partner if you have one, about one thing you'd enjoy sexually or about how a quick solo sex toy session helps you get off to sleep. For some people that's easy, but for the majority that would be a nightmare.

And that's exactly what The Hotbed Collective would like to change. One orgasm at a time.

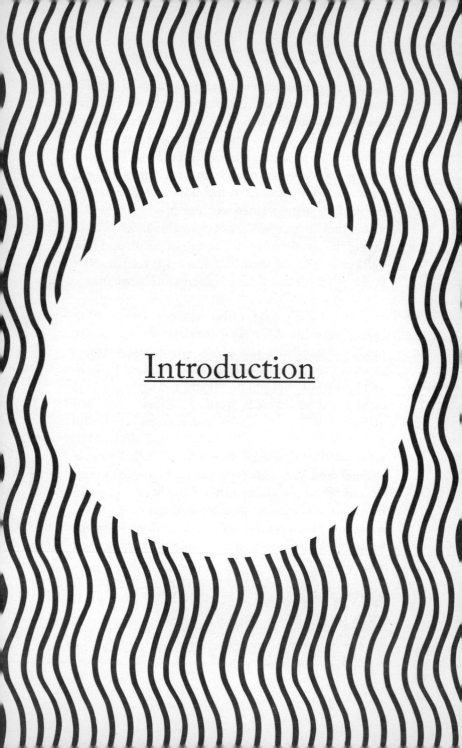

Introduction

There were many reasons not to write this book. What would Auntie Liz think? Would it embarrass our kids when they learn how to google us? Is it correct to offer our opinion on what women should do with their bodies? Is it even valid to talk about 'women' now that more people understand that the lines between 'women' and 'men' are not so clear-cut?

We set up our podcast *The Hotbed*, which launched on Valentine's Day 2018, because we'd become interested in the topic of sex in long-term relationships. And the more we talked about sex, the more women were telling us that *their* pleasure simply wasn't 'a priority', or that, while they enjoyed sex, their pleasure was not straight-forward and that it sometimes felt as though it was just not worth the effort: empowered, kickass women, who demanded equality in all other areas, accepted the dominance of male pleasure as the status quo.

> *That's just the way it is. It doesn't matter. It's not like I don't enjoy it.*

And so on …

While men mainly take their pleasure for granted, we're often putting up with boring sex. And while sex is boring, we're not going to initiate it. And when we don't initiate it – when we don't become agents of our own pleasure – our bodies and our voices are not equal. Relationships fizzle out. We feel anxious. We feel sad. And we can pay a fortune for quick-fix happiness solutions: new clothes, diet pills, holidays or … we could look a little closer to home. Just down there, between our legs.

An orgasm is a little, four-minute (or however long it takes) happy moment. It will help you sleep, keep you looking younger and, if you get it during partnered sex, help you feel closer to your partner and less likely to nag them about the Tupperware drawer. It is one of the things that can help relationships survive when the odds are stacked against them doing so. Orgasms are not a scarce resource. Orgasms are free and the good news is, having an orgasm doesn't take one away from someone else. It is not a zero sum game. The more orgasms the better, as far as we are concerned. In fact, we don't understand why there isn't more uproar about the fact that women are often having far fewer than men.

Although we were a little apprehensive about putting ourselves out there with *The Hotbed*, we quickly realised that the conversations we were starting were making other women feel happier, more normal and less alone. Very soon, we were getting emails that confirmed our own belief in the relevance of the podcast:

> *Thank you for starting this conversation ...*

> *Before your podcast, I had never heard of other women watching porn ...*

> *I feel better knowing that I'm not the only one who ...*

> *Listening to you made me realise something wasn't right with us ...*

> *My husband and I had a very hot night, thanks to you ...*

We were hearing from straight men too, who were also struggling for connection with their partners and wanting more mutual satisfaction and who were telling us that we were doing 'important work'. Dads who hadn't had sex in a long time and felt sad that they couldn't talk about it with their partners. Single women who were jaded by dating and looking for support.

We heard from bisexual women, from genderqueer and non-binary people who related to some of what we were saying, from older women who said they wished something like this had been around when they were eighteen.

We thought about Auntie Liz, and the awkward drinks party moments when someone asks us what we do for a living ... and, nevertheless, we concluded that we still wanted to carry on: educating, amplifying, normalising.

We also realised that we don't go to many drinks parties anyway.

The past couple of years have been bad for women and sex. Donald Trump and his boasts of 'pussy-grabbing', and the subsequent defence of this as 'boys will be boys' and 'locker room chat', appeared to put sexual relationships back into the Dark Ages. British broadcaster Piers Morgan, knowing what will boost ratings for his show *Good Morning Britain*, continues to dish out sexist crap such as 'has feminism gone too far?', whether he truly believes it or not.

The #MeToo movement has gained momentum, and women – and a few men – across the world are exposing their experience of sexual harassment and uniting their voices, and finding support and safety in numbers. The stories are difficult to read, but urgent and compelling, and we have a strong sense that change is afoot.

And as the #MeToo movement and its supporters work to take the shame away from victims of sexual abuse and sexual harassment, we want to help remove shame from the good kind of sex too. Sex that is consensual, fun and mutually satisfying. Sex with a partner, sex with yourself. We deserve sexual satisfaction as much as the next bloke. Why does it still feel radical to say that? Why isn't sexual pleasure a right and not a privilege for many women? What is getting in our way?

Our *raison d'être* is 'Making the world better, one orgasm at a time'. When we discussed this mission statement, however, we realised that even talking about orgasms still felt embarrassing for women. We worried that people would be put off by the book title and think that we were encouraging swinging parties and rubber nurses' uniforms for all. But what often hinders orgasm is not lack of kink, but lack of body confidence, and lack of positive sexual role models. Too often, we don't feel as if we deserve pleasure, and so we don't bother demanding change. It's easier not to – and it avoids an awkward conversation.

Admittedly, orgasm inequality isn't the biggest problem facing us today, but at least it's a relatively easy one to remedy. Having more orgasms isn't going to pollute the environment, or start a war – it's a tangible, meaningful, positive step in a world that often feels like it's gone completely bonkers. It's one which, with the right information and encouragement, we can take into our own hands (so to speak), and a woman in charge of her own sexuality is a formidable one.

We want to open those awkward conversations up, dispatch with the taboos, stop being so prudish and silly. We want to move the topic of the female orgasm beyond bawdy hen weekend chat and into the mainstream. Because why should a hen do be the only time we are legitimately allowed to talk about sex?

We believe that the more knowledge women have about their bodies, the less shame there is around how our bodies work — from hormones to periods to pelvic floors to pleasure. The more we know about our bodies, the more we know what gives us sexual satisfaction, what is and isn't right for *us*: we can express ourselves, speak out and, ultimately, enjoy life and all the stomach-jiggling, eye-opening and awe-inspiring experiences our body has to offer.

We were at an event recently when two women approached us. Woman One said, 'Oh, you're the Hotbed. I love you! I'm always telling people about you.' Woman One gestured towards Woman Two, 'She gets embarrassed about these things. She thinks I'm sex-mad.' Woman Two nodded and looked about as comfortable as someone who'd put her thong on back to front.

We were keen to talk to both women. Woman One is our ideal 'finished product': sex-positive, able to say what she likes, unembarrassed and killing it as a result. We hope she will read the book, nod furiously because it's what she thinks anyway, enthusiastically recommend it to colleagues and buy it for her friends, and maybe her mum and her teenage cousin.

But we also can relate to Woman Two.

We started *The Hotbed* from a position very much like that of Woman Two, and these are the people we would really like to reach as well: people who are capable of pleasure but who are shy of it. Those who loved sex at the beginning of a relationship but who feel the spark has gone. The ones who don't mind sex when it happens but who would rarely initiate it. The ones who may have masturbated a few times growing up, but rarely bother these days. Women who perhaps have put up with crap sex and feel sad that they're missing out.

These are our people! They are the way we also see ourselves. We are both women who feel like we could more boldly step out of our comfort zones. We haven't got it totally sussed but we want to feel as easy with our sexuality as many men do, and reap the rewards of regular orgasms (better sleep and better body image? Yes please).

What interests us too, is the reaction to our podcast from men.

Our first recording was in a sweaty downstairs bar in east London. We knew the crowd of women (mainly our friends) would be a bit shy about sharing their stories in public, so we handed out whistles and party horns so they could whistle or toot 'yes' or 'no' to our questions. Because Lisa was nine months pregnant and we were keen and naive and hoping to get everything in the bag before she went into labour, we recorded three episodes back to back. There was a lot of whistling, a lot of tooting, and a lot of sex information shared that night. By the end, some of the male bar staff looked a little shell-shocked. 'Wow, you ladies know how to drink,' one said. 'I wish I had heard all this before me and my girlfriend split up,' said another, looking a bit sad. We think he was referring to our discussion with our resident clinical psychologist and psychosexologist, Dr Karen Gurney, about female desire, during which we talked about how there is often more than meets the eye to a woman with a low sex drive (more on this below).

We hope that male readers will find *More Orgasms Please* enlightening. While we do complain about 'the patriarchy', we see this as the way our society currently works (with more men in decision-making positions, and more obstacles for women to reach the same), and not inherent in the actions and beliefs of all men: we believe that most men want their sexual partners to orgasm, and they would love more information on how to help them get there. This applies to women who have sex with women too.

This book is a combination of sex facts, practical advice, our personal stories and the odd detour into angry feminism. It will, we hope, arm women and their partners with useful tools and a wealth of information, and potentially also dispel a few unhelpful myths about women and their sexuality.

Women don't often feel the horn in a spontaneous and obvious way, as many men do, which is why lots of the time some of us might not be up for it or not feel very sexual (particularly when we have a big presentation to do the next morning or there's something really good on TV). We might worry about it and think our sex drive is low, or we might just conclude that it's not something we desperately need as much any more. 'Well, that was quite fun while it lasted but it's a *Radio Times* subscription that does it for me now, thanks very much!'

But, but, *but*: female desire is extremely responsive and, once we do decide to get it going (with a passionate kiss, an inner-thigh tickle, watching something sexy or engaging with a fantasy), it can go from zero to sixty very quickly. This is something most women and their partners would never know judging only by the kind of sex we see on screen.

But Hotbed, surely an orgasm is a nice-to-have rather than anything worth writing a book about?

Yeah, we get it: sex can be nice without the orgasm. Indeed, many women say they can enjoy sex regardless of whether they climax or not.

This book is definitely not designed to alienate anyone. We do not intend to make you feel embarrassed about the fact that you prefer making a nice stew to getting busy in the boudoir. (Although we'd guess that if you've bought this book you may have more than a passing interest in pursuing a more pleasure-filled existence.) There is enough pressure on us to be badass at work, on top of it all at home, to have a banging body and the latest-season clothes, that the last thing we want is to add yet another task to a busy woman's to-do list. We do, however, like the thought of the following:

TODAY'S GOALS

☐ **Call plumber**

☐ **Skype call at midday**

☐ **Finish tax return**

☐ **Hen-party hotel payment**

☐ **Change cat litter**

☐ **Have an orgasm**

Similarly, ever since we started The Hotbed Collective with several rounds of drinks, an Instagram account and twenty followers, we haven't made a habit of asking people about how *often* they masturbate and how *often* they have sex.

We know how bloody annoying to have to listen to someone wax lyrical about what a brilliant sex life they have. There is nothing worse than hearing a girlfriend recount how frequently she's having sex and feeling isolated and on the back foot ('God, my boyfriend can't keep his hands off me. We do it about three times a night').

It's important to remind yourself that everyone is different. What may feel like a lack in one person's life might be just fine, thank you, for another. It's *horses for courses*. But if you feel like you're not having enough sex or the kind of sex you want, then you're not. Conversely, perhaps you are having more sex than you feel you want or need. We heard from women who said that they are having sex because in some way they feel they owe it to their partners. This isn't satisfactory either.

There isn't an official number of times per month that you need to have sex in order to have a functioning relationship. So, it could be once every six months, three times a month or twice a week: it's about you and what feels right for you and your partner if you have one. We don't think it's helpful either to think of sex in terms of *quotas* and *targets* because desire doesn't work like that. Sex isn't like fruit and veg and making sure that you have your recommended '5 a day'. It's less about quantity and all about the quality of your sexual life; it's not about how often you have sex, nor is it all about how many orgasms you have, but we do want you to be in a position where you can have them if you want to, and to show you how to get there.

What we are advocating is that when you are having sex, that that sex is rewarding: for your pleasure to be the fullest and best it can be; to inspire you to feel curious and empower you to try different things; to treat your sex life as an extension of your life as a whole, and to live it to the full. Sex is one of the most enriching life experiences and the reality is we're deluged in sexual imagery but we don't always seem to be living sexy lives. So, just as you might have ambitions to write a book or visit Japan, so you might also want to try cunnilingus more often. In this sense, think of this book like a 'Couch to 5k' for your genitals.

Each chapter contains some suggestions of things you can try at home to achieve your goal, and you will find References and Resources sections at the end of the book which list useful reading and places to find extra help and information.

As well as being informative, we hope it will make you laugh. In an interview with the Spice Girls for *Vogue* magazine, American sex-positive writer Kathy Acker wrote that British feminism works by 'transforming society as society is best transformed, with lightness and in joy'. We agree. Laughter also releases feel-good endorphins and those endorphins help to release testosterone, which helps us feel hornier. It's a happy chain of events.

We want you to feel secure in the knowledge that you're having the kind of sex you want. And then, when it comes to partnered sex, you can tell your partner what turns you on, maybe even have the confidence to say that having your nipple bitten or being told 'I'm going to fuck you so hard your gash hurts' has always been a major turn-off and you want them to stop.

When you're feeling stressed and depleted, or in need of some ME-time, you might choose to give yourself an orgasm rather than shopping online, obsessively browsing Instagram or reading the *Daily Mail* sidebar of shame (and feeling like your soul is being sucked out via your eyeballs). You may do all of these things when the time is right (we do), but why not let having an orgasm remind you that constant consumption and comparison probably isn't the thing that lights the furnace of happiness that lives inside us all.

AN IMPORTANT NOTE ...

It's estimated that fewer than five per cent of women find it impossible to orgasm. It could be due to injury, disability or a gynaecological condition. Medication such as antidepressants and the contraceptive pill can sometimes affect arousal. Perhaps there has been a history of sexual abuse or past trauma which makes orgasm with a partner more difficult than alone. Equally, there is a small percentage of women with anorgasmia who are otherwise well. You may have once experienced an orgasm and then they've stopped. Or you may never have had one. You may care, or you may not. You may certainly have a wonderful sex life regardless. Orgasms are wonderful, but they are not *everything*, nor are they the sole merit of sex, and many of the benefits of an orgasm can be achieved through alternative sexual or physical activity.

We throw our hands up here to say that this book is not the place to find analysis of anorgasmia. We are not qualified and would rather direct you to people who are. The Resources section at the back lists some good sources of information and further help (the good news is that most cases of anorgasmia are treatable).

That is not to say that we haven't got your back. For us, orgasms are a convenient shorthand for wider issues such as body confidence, being able to explore fantasy and understanding our bodies a bit more. Everyone is entitled to a fully realised sexual identity, whatever shape that takes.

In the course of our research in writing *More Orgasms Please*, we read as many books, articles and studies about sexuality as we could lay our hands on. We interviewed experts, and dug deep into our own histories. Our findings and opinions in the pages that follow are based on what we have learnt in this process, and on two surveys which we have carried out ourselves.

The first was a survey of 700 people in which the respondents filled out an online questionnaire about sex after kids. The second was another online survey into female sexual pleasure which was completed by another 1,200 people. Both surveys, from a research point of view, were qualitative exercises, in that we tried to keep it as wide open as possible to get as many different experiences coming back to us. We make no claims for the scientific validity of the surveys we conducted. However, inspired by one of our heroines, Nancy Friday (more on her later), we decided that we would trust women to share their experiences honestly under the safety of anonymity, that we would take their answers in good faith, and use them to advance our understanding of female sexuality.

While our reading and research has been thorough, we will say, however, that not only is there still insufficient published scientific research into female sexual pleasure, but also that what is published is largely US-focused and concentrates predominantly on cis-women. We have included some references to trans women and trans men, both of whom have interesting stories to tell and as much right to sexual pleasure as the next person.

That said, there is undoubtedly a bias in this book which we would like to acknowledge, and recognise that some trans folk may find parts of the book, by its very nature, and with its references to anatomy, gender dysphoric.

We didn't want this book to feel like some old-school instructional manual and we hope you won't find that reading it is like sitting down to homework. For that reason, we don't talk about pregnancy or sexually-transmitted diseases (the current mainstay of sex ed). We do however, want you to feel free to skip some chapters if they're not up your street or you'd like to come back to them later.

We'd also love to suggest couples read it together and use it as the starting point for a conversation about sex, but we also know this sounds very *Joy of Sex*-like: perhaps it was excruciating for you to even read this idea. Panic not. Maybe, instead, women in relationships could leave this book open at key pages so their partners might have a read, or put it in their loo so a partner and visitors can read it while they're in there, or leave it on the bus, thus giving the general public some secrets to female orgasms in between stops.

Sex is the universal leveller. Most of us do it at some stage. We fret that we aren't doing it as much/as well as other people. You might be inspired to chat to a couple of your mates about our book and it will hopefully open up some honest and perhaps helpful conversations, and talking about sex is massive fun, as we've discovered from our podcasts and from researching and writing this book.

One last thing: we should acknowledge here that for some of us, having an orgasm — particularly if it's something we may not have prioritised until now — can require a bit of dedicated time and application. Even at its most mechanical, an orgasm is something which requires some input from your mind as well as your body. We assure you that practising and trying out some of the tips we will give in the following chapters will at least be fun, and the effort is *worth it*.

What Exactly Is an Orgasm?

1

LISA

I'm seventeen and in bed with my boyfriend. Green-eyed, olive-skinned and a gifted bass player, he is studying at the university near to where I live. We met on Valentine's Day in our local nightclub about fifteen minutes after I'd vomited my dinner and four cocktails into one of those free-standing ashtrays (classy). Although we don't have a huge amount in common, our conversation can stretch just about long enough to get next to each other on his single bed and start kissing. As The Man Who *by Travis plays on in the background, the action heats up until our hands are everywhere, clothes are removed, a condom applied and he's on top of me. I run my hands down his back as he takes a thrust. About seven minutes later, maybe ten, he says:*

'I'm about to come, how far off are you?'

I have no idea how to answer. I'd given myself a couple of orgasms before but I'd never managed it during intercourse and, as attractive as I find him, I'm fairly sure I'm not about to start here. But, in the heat of the moment, how do you find the words to say this? How do you find the words to say this at any time? He'd take it personally, he'd think there was something wrong with me (and I'm beginning to think there is), and the whole situation is so awkward I'd almost prefer to have let out a huge fanny fart than to have to answer this question. After a minute of inner cringing, I say I don't know, say we can stop, and then kiss him with such 'passion' that he can't ask me any more questions. As I gather my stuff up to leave, the Travis LP is still playing in the background.

Travis aside, we're pretty sure that the scenario Lisa describes is happening in bedrooms all over the world. Most men take their pleasure for granted. Many women don't. And if we are hoping for an orgasm the way we see them happen on screen (a few thrusts and we're there), when we don't 'come', we feel awkward, inadequate. And it's so hard to talk about — is it shame? Is it because we don't have the words? Is it because we don't want to disappoint or upset someone? — that we might overcompensate with extra kisses (so no one can talk), or divert attention away from the awkwardness by talking about sandwiches, or Sainsburys. Or Syria, even? Just definitely not the sex. Anything but the sex.

Life is too short for bad sex. It's too short for awkward non-conversations, for avoiding sex because you know it's not that fun, or for having to drink yourself silly before you allow yourself to let go. It's too short not to love your body, or not to know some really interesting things about it.

So, let's start with some basics. Like, what exactly is an *orgasm*?

An orgasm is defined by the *Oxford English Dictionary* as:

> *The climax of sexual excitement, character-ised by intensely pleasurable feelings centred in the genitals and (in men) experienced as an accompaniment to ejaculation.*

According to the *OED*, the origin is 'Late 17th century: from French *orgasme*, or from modern Latin *orgasmus*, from Greek *orgasmos*, from organ *"swell or be excited"*.'

Woohoo, we're already excited! Particularly as we know that the swelling is not just the preserve of the male orgasm, and neither is the ejaculation. Women can swell, women can ejaculate.

Women's orgasms can be any number of things and they can vary from woman to woman, and from orgasm to orgasm. That's partly what makes them so wonderful. But a female orgasm is generally accepted to include some or all of the following:

• Intense pleasure
• Feeling of release
• Raising of the heartbeat
• Shortening of the breath
• Natural lubrication of the vagina and/or a gland near the urethra, including what can be referred to as an ejaculation
• Contracting of the vaginal muscles

Orgasms in women are a combination of physical and mental and environmental factors. From a physical point of view, while sensitive areas such as nipples, thighs and the anus can play a role in climax, it happens predominantly as a result of stimulation to the tip or the 'head' of the clitoris (the pea-sized bump towards the top of the vulva – more on this in chapter 4). Some women (around twenty per cent) can also orgasm through vaginal stimulation (either inter-course or with a finger/sex toy).

Many women feel as if not coming through intercourse means there is something wrong with them. There isn't. It's actually pretty damn normal. In fact, if you don't reach orgasm during vaginal intercourse alone, you're in the majority: the eighty per cent. We need to get that out the way now because, in our experience, it is one of the most eye-opening and normalising facts about female pleasure.

We included a number of specific questions about orgasms in our survey on female pleasure, so, to get us in the mood, here are some descriptions of what it feels like for a girl, submitted kindly by some of the 1,200 respondents to our questionnaire:

> *It starts from the clitoris and spreads through into my abdomen with pulsating contractions that speed up and then slow down. It feels like it lasts a lot longer than it probably does in real time. I'm not aware of thinking anything after 'here we go'. It sometimes feels like warmth spreading through my abdomen, but not always.*

> *Clitoris, uterus and anus throb and flutter. My legs go stiff, then wobbly. My chest goes red. Sometimes I ejaculate.*

> *Some orgasms, when rushed, feel less intense and as soon as I feel it come on, I know that it's a 'shallow' low-level orgasm ... that kind of annoys me. The best ones start deep inside, in my legs, and travel up into my groin but it feels really deep and intense and, a lot of the time, I see flickers of light in my vision as soon as I reach climax ... my heart races like hell*

and all I want is for the feeling to last longer than it does !! #greedy, haha.

With some orgasms, I can feel it in my head: they make me fuzzy and inarticulate. Some are just quick spasms and then finished.

It's like it almost fills up my whole body, reaches a crescendo and then the feeling turns into bliss — like you're being carried on water/ clouds. My mind completely switches off, and I'm in the moment totally.

We were thrilled to read the descriptions of orgasms from our survey; there was something so beautiful hearing about pleasure in women's own words. In many ways an orgasm is indescribable, but we think our respondents came very close and out of the responses some common themes emerged:

- A sense of being out-of-body

- A feeling and sensation beyond the vulva area: many women mentioned toes, stomach, legs and breasts

- A feeling of such intense pleasure that, when it's happening, they feel they want another orgasm immediately (which is how we feel when we eat a chocolate Hobnob, incidentally)

- A feeling of soft, natural movement such as 'waves' or 'clouds'

We also asked which words best described their orgasms. We offered some examples, but also left a space for them to add their own adjectives and these are just some of the responses on the following page.

What's interesting is that, though their equipment may be different and though women have a much shorter period of downtime between orgasms (known as the 'refractory period'), meaning they are much more likely to be able to have multiple orgasms (another great score for the sisterhood), men and women are thought to experience orgasms in a similar way. The pleasure is equal, the physical responses are similar, and both get a little boost of oxytocin (the 'love hormone' which makes you feel close to the person you just came with), which all goes to show that deep down we're not all that different after all.

'GOOD SEX IS LIKE GOOD BRIDGE. IF YOU DON'T HAVE A GOOD PARTNER, YOU'D BETTER HAVE A GOOD HAND.'

Mae West

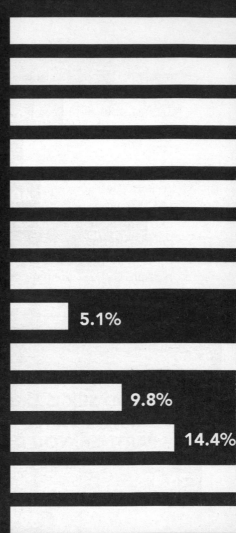

electric

thrilling

exciting

hot

thumping

primal

energising

mystical 5.1%

out-of-body

surreal 9.8%

wild 14.4%

nice

moreish

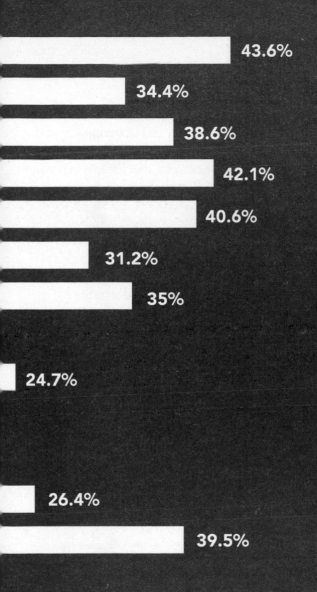

43.6%

34.4%

38.6%

42.1%

40.6%

31.2%

35%

24.7%

26.4%

39.5%

WHICH WORDS WOULD YOU USE TO DESCRIBE YOUR ORGASMS?

1,191 responses

WHY DO WE ORGASM?

There would be no babies without male orgasms. Men need to climax in order to procreate, and so boring sex for men might lead to a big drop in the fertility rate and, eventually, render us extinct as a species, leaving behind just a few of our skeletons hanging in the Natural History Museum. And Cher.

But why do women orgasm? Is it just so there's something in it for us as an incentive to help populate the earth? Quite a few theories have been tested, and they are all explained, and, one by one, discredited, by Professor Elizabeth Lloyd in her book *The Case of the Female Orgasm*. The theory we found the most outlandish was that female orgasm originated as a way of making sure that it wasn't just the alpha male of a pack who got all the girls (as well as all the hunting spoils and the cave with the best view). With the remaining males able to drive the women wild with their sexy moves, bonding could happen, and men would get some sugar and therefore be motivated to get up every day and hunt a crust. The tribe would stay together, grow and ultimately survive.

Professor Lloyd thinks that the truth is a little less convoluted: she believes that female orgasms are a happy by-product of the fact that, in embryo, what becomes a penis in a boy and a vulva in a girl starts off as the same thing (more on this later). Whatever the explanation is for our orgasms, though, we'll take it. Thank you very much.

DO ORGASMS MATTER?

Female orgasms are hot – for the women experiencing them, and for their partners. Why wouldn't we want more? Women who are having better sex, more masturbation and more orgasms sleep better, have a greater sense of wellbeing and are able to use this energy in other areas of their lives. Scientific studies over the years have found that female sexual satisfaction can have the following results:

• Increased continence (i.e. better bladder control)

• Better skin quality

• A more youthful appearance (this sounds like marketing BS but we promise you, the evidence is there)

• Strengthens your immune system

• Bonds you to your sexual partner

• Decreased risk of heart disease

• Even more orgasms (having a good sex life leads to a better sex life because just as you can train to be good at swimming, you can effectively 'train' your body to be good at sex)

So far so good, yet reading the responses in our survey, we were interested to note another recurring theme: many women reported a feeling of shame or embarrassment either after orgasm, or around writing about it. Many respondents mentioned that before answering our questions they had never thought too much about the subject, let alone written about it, and some said that they just didn't have the words.

The picture becomes more troubling when we consider the latest research into orgasm inequality: a 2017 study which looked at the sex lives of more than 50,000 Americans found that ninety-five per cent of straight men nearly or always have an orgasm when they have sex, compared to eighty-nine per cent of gay men, eighty-eight per cent of bisexual men and eighty-six per cent of lesbians. Then comes **THE GAP**: only sixty-six per cent of bisexual women said they always or nearly always orgasm when they are sexually intimate with someone else, and sixty-five per cent of heterosexual women.

Similar studies, including our own survey, have returned slightly different percentages but the same proportions. Whichever way one looks at it, there's an orgasm gap — and women are losing out. It is our belief that closing this gap matters — a lot. The fact that there is such a stark gender divide, and within it also one of sexual orientation, suggests to us that there is a problem not only with how we view and provide for women in society, but also with how women and men interact with each other on a sexual and emotional level.

A Public Health England (PHE) survey in 2018 of more than 7,000 women found that forty-nine per cent of women aged between twenty-five and thirty-four (also the age group making up the majority of *The Hotbed*'s audience) were dissatisfied with their sex life. In addition, fifty-one per cent of all the women surveyed said that in the previous year they had experienced one or more sexual difficulties (such as lack of sexual enjoyment, menstrual issues or incontinence) lasting more than *three months*, and less than half of these women sought help for these problems, regardless of severity. Having compiled that report (which also took into account issues such as infertility, menopause, period poverty and sexual abuse), PHE concluded that the poor state of women's reproductive health was a public health issue, much like smoking, dementia and air pollution.

Sexual difficulties in women leading to the orgasm gap, we believe, are in no small part a consequence of how we educate our children, how we represent women and sex in the media, on screen and in porn, how badly many women feel about their bodies, how little we all know about our anatomy, and how talking about sex and pleasure can be about as easy as poking yourself in the eye with a barbecue skewer.

We're not the first people to point this out. In 1976 Shire Hite published her findings from asking 3,000 women to talk about their sex lives. She found the same trends as we did: that a huge number of heterosexual women, who had no trouble orgasming when they masturbated, were not reaching the same climax when they had sex with men. She blamed culture and not biology, saying we need to redefine what sex is and not accept it as simply a bit of foreplay, then intercourse until the man comes. She likened this status quo to a form of 'sexual slavery', writing:

> *Women are sexual slaves in so far as they are (justifiably) afraid to 'come out' with their own sexuality, and forced to satisfy others' needs and ignore their own. As one woman put it, 'sex can be political in the sense that it can involve a power structure where the woman is unwilling or unable to get what she really needs for her fullest amount of pleasure, but the man is getting what he wants, and the woman, like an unquestioning and unsuspecting lackey, is gratefully supplying it'.*

Has much changed since 1976?

Has it fuck.

HOW LONG DOES IT NORMALLY TAKE YOU TO REACH ORGASM DURING MASTURBATION?

1,183 responses

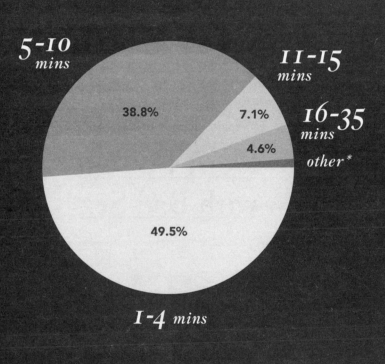

5-10 *mins* — 38.8%

11-15 *mins* — 7.1%

16-35 *mins* — 4.6%

other*

1-4 *mins* — 49.5%

* including those who said they don't masturbate or have never had an orgasm. We also asked how long it took to come to orgasm during parterned sex and the most popular answer was 5-10 minutes (38.5%) followed by 11-15 minutes (29.7%).

Don't Put Up
with Bad Sex

2

ANNIKI

It's the late Eighties. I'm fifteen. I've been out at a nightclub with a bunch of friends. We've drunk Grolsch, and been chatted up by some students from St Martin's School of Art. They are channelling the Levi's 501 ads and wear white T-shirts and baggy jeans.

One of them asks if I want to go back to his room. My best friend Hannah accompanies me. He lives in a hall of residence in Battersea. To cut a long story short, the boy and I snog while Hannah sleeps in the same bed. This is not unusual as beds are often at a premium and we've become used to sharing this way. Without warning the boy clambers on top of me and starts thrusting. Hannah mumbles, 'Can you please stop?' but the boy continues.

Eventually after three minutes he groans. I am still wearing my thick Wolford tights. They must be at least 200 denier.

'You are completely gross,' Hannah says waking up. 'I'm getting out of here.'

I don't want to stay without her so we leave. On the early-morning bus up the King's Road, I look down at my tights. There is a white sticky substance. 'I can't believe you had sex in the bed next to me,' Hannah says.

The conversation ended right there. Had I had sex? Was that it? The problem was I lacked the necessary vocabulary to explain what had happened. My sex ed lessons hadn't included a session on 'dry humping'. 'Could I be pregnant?' I wondered. There were rumours that sperm was so powerful that it could survive outside your body and crawl up your leg if it was determined enough. I never talked about this experience with anyone — not even my best mate.

I also felt ashamed but wasn't quite sure why. There was no one I could talk to about it. I spent many hours fretting that my future sex life would be one where I always had sex through a pair of tights because I didn't know any better.

'Bad sex' experiences such as the one Anniki describes above unfortunately are the norm for many young women embarking on those first few formative sexual experiences. Without a meaningful, realistic idea of what to expect or useful education about how sex is supposed to be *pleasurable*, then it's a miracle that we ever end up enjoying it at all.

If you don't know your own anatomy, what a clitoris is, or the difference between foreplay and penetration, then *having sex through a pair of tights* can be the unfortunate outcome. Sex education lays the groundwork. It also encourages us to talk about our experiences so we don't think we're abnormal. It gives us the information we need to make the right choices (and these will hopefully lead to more orgasms and less worry, anxiety and ignorance).

Bad sex probably shares a few common traits (for us anyway).

FIRSTLY: no orgasm. Of course, you can have nice sex without an orgasm but if you are physically capable of an orgasm, it's a bit like eating rhubarb crumble without custard. Or not having a bun with your burger. Or going out with trainers and no socks so your feet get blisters (come up with your own analogy here). You can fake an orgasm (and sometimes it's just simply the easiest thing to do: if it's someone you haven't had sex with much yet and you like them but you haven't finished this book yet and are therefore still mid-journey to becoming a fully qualified sex goddess who can ask for what she likes) but this isn't a sustainable way forward and the sooner you can put things right, the better.

SECONDLY: bad sex often hurts. This may be because you're not lubricated enough and your sexual partner has no clue or has forgotten about foreplay, or because they've watched too much porn, and think frantic, crazy, Jack Russell-style action is what turns you on (maybe it does, in which case: thumbs up).

THIRDLY: bad sex sometimes entails something happening which is so humiliating that your face burns whenever you think about it, even when it's twenty-odd years later.

If you have good friends who have at some point talked to you about sex, you will almost certainly have heard stories about bad sex. If you haven't and all your friends have only ever had good sex, then please can you contact us via our publisher (address on the imprint page) and let us know their secrets?

We know from our own conversations and from feedback from *The Hotbed* that plenty of bad sex is happening each and every day. Here are some quick-fire stories about bad encounters, shared with us by our listeners:

> *The time I tried to give a blow job but thought you had to blow instead of suck …*

The time toilet paper was still stuck to my bum and I was really into a guy and he discovered it there ...

I had to pee really bad and ended up weeing all over our sleeping bag ...

My entire first relationship involved sex which was OK but which never made me have an orgasm ...

His mum rang him while we were at it, and he answered and had a full conversation with her before carrying on again ...

In *Not That Kind of Girl*, Lena Dunham describes a bad experience of cunnilingus: 'I felt like I was being chewed on by a child that wasn't mine.'

Author and columnist Caitlin Moran refers to bad sex as 'the straight-up awful hump – a tale you will tell for the rest of time'. She tells a story of going back to a famous comedian's house in the Nineties: 'As we began the "opening monologue" on the sofa, he reached around for the remote control – and put on his own TV show.'

Perhaps you too have your own bad sex story to tell. Often the accounts of these experiences share certain commonalities: we're disempowered, passive, naïve and insecure. We do something stupid and embarrassing and we don't have the guts to ride it out.

Our partner is too rough, not rough enough, too fast, too slow, rude, arrogant, or picks his toenails afterwards.

WHEN 'BAD SEX' CROSSES THE LINE, IT IS NOT ALL RIGHT

Bad sex, sex that makes you cringe or yawn when you think about it, is bad enough. There is another class of sex, however, that is never OK. Sex that is abusive and damaging, destructive and ego-destroying. Sex which makes you feel sick, unsafe, angry or sad. If this applies to you – and the latest statistics show that one in five women in the UK have experienced some kind of sexual abuse/assault – please consider seeking help with a professional who can give legal and medical advice and refer you for counselling and/or legal recourse. Everyone is entitled to sexual pleasure and help is available. (For a list of organisations offering support, see the Resources section on p.347.)

Samantha from *Sex and the City* famously declared, 'Fuck me badly once, shame on you. Fuck me badly twice, shame on me.' You will have noticed that we're not blaming our sexual partners exclusively for our bad sex. Of course, they should get clued up: read about some techniques; buy lube; ask you what you like and dislike; and know that women don't tend to get turned on by having their head forced down into the crotch area. But while they should be able to read your body language, they can't be expected to read your mind.

Bad sex can happen when expectations are running very high. It can happen when you're fifteen and it can happen when you're eighty-five. Unless women take responsibility for their own pleasure and get educated about what pleases them, and have the confidence to tell or show their partners, bad sex can last an entire lifetime.

HOW BAD SEX CAN HAVE A LONG-TERM IMPACT ON OUR SEXUALITY

It's well known that our formative years shape the way we feel about ourselves. The taunts about being overweight or the cousin who said you looked like a bloke; the boy who told you that your legs would be ace if you were a rugby player; or the fact that you never got picked for the netball team. Most of us have similar demons in our heads: the voices that say you're ugly, useless and your body is fucking awful can lead to feelings of low self-esteem and make us devalue ourselves and our right to feel pleasure.

Add to this the lack of a decent sex education, and the fact that there are so many myths about sex floating about, and it follows that we approach sex with low and fearful expectations. For Anniki it meant she started off scared of the penis because it was automatically linked to pregnancy.

There was no mention of pleasure. In reality most of us were masturbating but we wouldn't have talked to our friends about it. If nobody talks openly about sex, then bad sex will continue to fester in the background. If we can't talk to our friends and share our experiences, both good and bad, we probably will find it even harder to be assertive and broach the subject with our partners. Our expectations are lowered, bad patterns become entrenched and, unchecked, bad, unsatisfying sex then persists way beyond our teens and twenties.

Twenty-five years later Anniki asked her friend Hannah if she'd masturbated when they were teenagers. Hannah had to leave the room for a couple of minutes. 'Of course I bloody did,' she replied on her return.

Did you ever talk to your friends about masturbation? Do you talk about it now? What about talking to your daughters? Do you raise them so they know that masturbation is their right if they want it? That it's nothing to be ashamed of? Do you arm them with the information they need so they don't ever settle for sex through a pair of tights?

The sad thing is, things aren't necessarily changing for the better today. Yes, there's more in terms of seeing sex on screen but now, if anything, girls have too many preconceptions of what sex should look and feel like, and they're often learning from porn without knowing that porn is a fantasy and not a tutorial video.

Talking about porn in the modern age, Peggy Orenstein, author of *Girls & Sex,* points out that:

> *forty-one per cent of videos (porn) included 'ass to mouth' in which, immediately after removing his penis from a woman's anus, he places it in her mouth. Scenes of 'bukkake sex' (multiple men ejaculating on a woman's face), 'facial abuse' (oral sex aimed at making a woman vomit), triple penetration and penetration by multiple penises in a single orifice are also on the rise. I'm going to go out on a limb here and say that in real life those practices wouldn't feel good to most women.*

Previous generations of women have been disadvantaged because they knew too little and were exposed to so little sex on screen or in the media, that they had limited means to find out about what they wanted. On the plus side, we had our imaginations and our partners were usually green as well. Now women are more enlightened in terms of seeing lots of sex, lots of a certain type of sex, but are limited by what the dominant male ideology tells them is sexy. Things that weren't normalised before have become more commonplace — and some of these things simply don't *feel good.*

We have to rewrite our own sexual narratives so that sex is more empowering and pleasurable and ensure that the next generation gets the right messages too.

Orenstein outlines what needs to change:

> *I recently suggested to a friend of mine, a woman who, like me is a feminist ... that it was not enough to teach our daughters about the mechanics of reproduction, not enough to encourage resistance to unwanted sexual pressure. It was not enough to equip them with birth control pills and condoms ... We needed to talk to them about good sex, starting with how their own bodies worked, with masturbation and orgasm.*

It's about talking to a generation who are growing up with more than a torn page from a porn mag or a well-thumbed sexy extract from a Jackie Collins novel. It's vitally important that young women share their experiences and learn from them. It's about discussing female pleasure and how good sex isn't just about avoiding pregnancy. It's about mobilising and empowering women so they are unafraid to talk about sex and the things that bring them pleasure. It definitely feels like the right time for this to happen: the younger generation are already redefining identity politics and we need to see the same thing happen for sex.

On a more personal level, however, how can we move on from bad sex? The he-shagged-me-through-my-tights sex, the he-watched-TV-while-we-were-doing-it sex, the sex that makes you want to join a nunnery, or at least buy a *Handmaid's Tale* outfit and avoid eye contact with anyone you might find attractive. This isn't just about young women being better informed and more confident in their sexuality, it's also about older generations stepping up to the plate and shaking off their old, negative sexual histories and reclaiming their right to pleasure.

Here's our Hotbed advice:

REMEMBER IT'S NEVER TOO LATE TO REWRITE YOUR SEXUAL STORY. Just as we can change jobs and have multiple identities, so we can change the course of our sexual history. Have a frank look at your own sex life — look at the overarching narrative from teen to now. What percentage has been bad? Are there any patterns in terms of things you've put up with but would rather not any more? How can you build on the stuff you love?

THINK ABOUT THE BEST SEX YOU'VE HAD AND WHAT SHAPED THOSE EXPERIENCES. Was it a specific technique? A mood? Location? It might not be possible to recreate a summer in Spain when you were twenty-two, but there will be certain ingredients that you can integrate into your sex life now …

GET OVER THE IDEA THAT SEX IS BEST WHEN YOU'RE YOUNG. The reality is often quite the opposite. The Public Health England survey that we referred to earlier found that forty-two per cent of women aged between twenty-five and thirty-four complained of 'a lack of sexual enjoyment', but in the fifty-five to sixty-four age group this percentage falls to twenty-eight per cent (more on this in chapter 16: Growing Old Disgracefully). Bad sex can be edifying in that it teaches you what you *don't* want from a sexual encounter, meaning you can learn and improve as you grow older (despite the media's failure to portray any woman past thirty as fuckable).

TAP INTO FANTASY. When we're younger we have rich fantasy lives. Usually these take the shape of imagining sex with pop stars and actors. How can fantasy help now? How can you tap into that teen mindset where sex lived in your imagination? (If you need some more help, we have a chapter on fantasy coming up, as it happens).

OF COURSE IT MAY BE EASIER TO FAKE IT TILL YOU MAKE IT, ESPECIALLY DURING NEW ENCOUNTERS, BUT THERE'S NO REASON WHY YOU CAN'T HAVE GREAT SEX WHILE DATING HOT STRANGERS. Showing someone where and how you liked to be touched, bringing along a tube of lube, and saying 'softer', 'this is amazing,' or 'ooh, that hurts a bit', are all completely acceptable from the first bonk, and could spare you both some embarrassment and wasted time.

OWN YOUR BAD SEX STORIES. Talk about them. You'll soon discover that they're pretty much universal. A bad sex story shared is a bad sex story out in the open and you can have a good old hoot about it and relieve yourself of any shame. We're talking about the sex-through-tights stories here, of course. If they're about anything abusive or damaging in any shape or form then seek help from a counsellor or therapist. The experience of abuse can't be brushed under the carpet and will oftentimes leave heavy imprints in your memory, but with proper support and therapy they don't have to be a barrier to improving your sex life either.

Bad sex may be a rite of passage but as we've explained, it can also continue from our teens into our twenties, thirties and beyond. There may no longer be Wolford tights involved, but there will certainly be times when your partner can't perform, or you lose interest, or the baby cries, or you're too tired, or the quality of sex is *just not there* for you.

In order to stop the rot and make sure that it's not happening *all the time*, look out for unhelpful patterns that emerge. Do you always tend to prioritise your partner's pleasure more than your own? Do you feel grateful if your partner makes your orgasm a priority but then worry afterwards that you were being too demanding and pushy? Do you cringe when you tell your partner about what turns you on?

It's also worth remembering that famous Nora Ephron quote about how you can turn embarrassing stories around so you become the heroine: 'When you slip on a banana peel, people laugh at you. But when you tell people you slipped on a banana peel, it's your laugh.' That's how Anniki feels about the whole tights story anyway. She's 'owning' that bad boy.

TOP WOMEN (AND ONE MAN) WHO GIVE US SEXUAL CONFIDENCE

(and when to channel their sexual energy)

Who are the women that inspire you the most?

Do you ever look at some women and think **GOD, IT SERIOUSLY LOOKS LIKE SHE'S NOT AFRAID TO ASK FOR WHAT SHE WANTS?**

Don't you wish that you could channel some of that sexual chutzpah? Sometimes all we need are some positive female role models who live their positive sexual lives, who we can look up to and go, 'Yeah, she wouldn't put up with crappy sex or shame herself out of masturbating.'

Courtney Love

Courtney Love is the lead singer of the band Hole and partner of the late Kurt Cobain. Back in the day, she was vilified in the media for being out of control, and dressing inappropriately. But at *The Hotbed* we think she's a powerful, sexy woman who knows how to shake up a room. Take a leaf out of Courtney's book whenever you're in need of a good kick up the arse.

FAVOURITE HOTBED COURTNEY-ISM: 'Jack White,

you're worthy of my p**sy. He's a classicist, he's confident, he carries himself well.'

WHEN TO CHANNEL COURTNEY: On a boring Saturday night when *The Voice* is on the telly, you've just eaten a takeaway and need to switch things up a bit. At Pizza Express during an all-too-predictable birthday celebration.

Grace Jones

If you're worried about the age-lines forming around your eyes, we recommend googling Grace Jones's 2012 performance of 'Slave to the Rhythm' at the Queen's Jubilee celebrations (which makes it all the more sur-real). Grace sports a red rubber corset, a headdress and keeps a giant hula hoop gyrating the whole time. Grace is now seventy years old.

FAVOURITE HOTBED GRACE-ISM: 'Pull up to my bumper baby, in your long, black limousine.'

WHEN TO CHANNEL GRACE: When someone has just pointed out that you look like you haven't slept in six months. At a wedding. At the swimming pool in your new Asos swimming costume.

Madonna

Say what you like about her — oh, and people do, how they do — but Madonna was a visible sexually empowered role model for many girls growing up in the eighties and Nineties. She was rude and honest about sex and relationships. She wasn't afraid to express her sexuality. Songs like 'Express Yourself', and 'Justify My Love' always put her at the forefront of the sexual zeitgeist, let alone the film *In Bed with Madonna* in which she demonstrated how to give a blow job to a generation of horny teenagers.

FAVOURITE HOTBED MADONNA-ISM: 'I don't want to be your Mother. I don't want to be your sister either. I just want to be your lover.'

WHEN TO CHANNEL MADONNA: On a first date. On a second date.

Kate Bush

Kate Bush is one of those women who is so influential that even boring old, muso-farts who think they're the only people who lived through the punk era drone on about her for hours on BBC4, and endlessly hypothesise about the true meaning behind her music. The truth is, Kate Bush is a BADASS. She deserves an entire book devoted to her genius as a feminist icon. An amazing songwriter, talented dancer *and* performer, she has remained a sexual enigma (hence lots of old music journalists hypothesising themselves into a right old state of excitement). She has a sexual energy that is dark, pagan and reminds us of strange fairy creatures who lived in trees in medieval England.

FAVOURITE HOTBED KATE-ISM: 'Here I go. It's coming for me through the trees. Help me someone, help me please ...' (Is Kate fleeing her own rampant, sexual longing? Oh look, now we're hypothesising.)

WHEN TO CHANNEL KATE BUSH: At a festival. At the Halloween party.

Amber Rose

We first noticed Amber Rose at the MTV Music Video Awards in 2009. She has a shaved head, and a face that is almost soothing to look at. Her then boyfriend Kanye West hopped on stage to bang on about Beyoncé when Taylor Swift won Best Video, and though we couldn't see Amber's reaction, we're pretty sure it would have been *eyeroll*. Amber went on to be one of the most high-profile sex-positive campaigners in the US. She has a sex podcast called *Loveline* and every year hosts a slutwalk to make the point that, no matter how you act or dress, you do not 'deserve' to be sexually assaulted.

FAVOURITE HOTBED AMBER-ISM: 'If a grown mother-of-two is comfortable with her body and wants to show it off, that's none of your business or anyone else's.'

WHEN TO CHANNEL AMBER: On a date night. Most weekends.

Buck Angel

Very much not a woman but we wanted to include trans activist Buck, who describes himself as a 'man with a female past' because he is so in charge of his own sexuality and is so encouraging of others. He uses Instagram to champion self-acceptance, to answer questions about sex tools for those with vaginas (including his own 'Buck Off' sex toy) and to be a massive legend, generally. Even if you are not a trans man, his words will make you feel the love, we promise, especially when he signs off all his posts with an affectionate 'Tranpa'.

FAVOURITE BUCK-ISM: 'Genital shame has been handed down for a very long time. Vagina shame! It's fucking real. I then think to myself how lucky I am to have learned to embrace my vagina as a man. To show the world with no fear.'

WHEN TO CHANNEL BUCK: When you want to say 'buck off' to any embarrassment or shame about your body, identity or sexuality.

And finally …

Channel Yourself

We're not getting all Oprah here, but think back to a time when you felt like you really had it GOING ON. It might have been a night out. Or at an event. Your honeymoon. Anything. Now try and think back to the things that made you feel sexually confident and with it. Channel that energy. Remember that you've felt sexy and will feel sexy again. Channel yourself.

WHAT FACTORS CONTRIBUTED TO YOU NOT HAVING AN ORGASM DURING PARTNERED SEX IN THE PAST YEAR?

1,195 responses

58.8%
Not feeling aroused prior to sex

41%
Poor body image

40.3%
Feeling rushed by time constraints

35.1%
Mental health

31.2%
Not being able to communicate desires/preferences with partner

31%
Feeling rushed by partner

27.8%
Other worries

Respondents could tick as many boxes as applied. Other factors included lack of skill of partner, feeling too cold and feeling unclean/unhygienic.

How Lit Is
Your Clit?

3

LISA

The first time I heard the word 'clitoris' was when Ellen DeGeneres said it. I was thirteen and watching late-night TV. It was during a stand-up routine about sex, and she talked about what a funny word it is, and how your tongue sticks out a bit when you say it and so, if you say 'clitoris' enough times while performing oral sex on a woman, you could make them have an orgasm. I could gather, by association, that the 'clitoris' must be somewhere near your vagina, because I knew that was where the rude stuff happened. But back then, I wouldn't have been very familiar or comfortable even with the word 'vagina'. I would have read it in a biology textbook, but I never used the word.

I never talked about 'that area' and I never touched it, unless I had to. I knew Robbie Williams's favourite word (funky) but I didn't know what a clitoris was. I knew that Kevin from the Backstreet Boys' nickname was Train ('Because I'm always rushing around ...') but I would have referred to my vulva as 'my bottom' or, if I needed to make myself clear, 'my ... front bottom'.

I knew that Keanu meant 'cool breeze' in Hawaiian, but when I read a Judy Blume book called Deenie *and the main character talked about touching her 'special place' until she felt better, I pressed down on my wrist quite hard and wondered why nothing happened.*

Not only is 'clitoris' a great word which, if you say it over and over while performing oral sex on a woman, could make her have an orgasm, but it is a great organ too. Judy Blume was right, it really is a special place: packed with nerve endings which, when manoeuvred in the right way, can make our legs shake and our vaginas wet, and fill our head with stars. The clitoris is so amazing, it is a mystery to us why there aren't entire shrines dedicated to it, why there isn't an entire line of clitoris-shaped novelty items (cake tins, party hats, piñatas) on sale in Ann Summers, and why there aren't as many architecturally perfect buildings fashioned in their image as there are boob-like domes and phallic skyscrapers (we don't think there's even one).

There are a few clit-shaped glimmers of hope in this world. Look up 'clitoris' on craft marketplace Etsy and you'll find several pages of artisan goods in its image: from sparkly earrings to a wine stopper. Download the OMGYes! app, which lets you touch a screen to master clitoris-pleasing techniques. At £49, it's expensive for an app but, as Emma Watson says, 'it's worth it' (and often there are half-price deals. Even those most orgasmic among us love a bargain). Find enlightened publications such as *Bustle*, *Cosmopolitan*, the *Guardian* and *Refinery29* writing on the topic. Follow the artist Clitorisity on Instagram. She makes a habit of chalking up pavements with clitoris-shaped graffiti with captions such as 'Do you know what this is?' It's a piss in the ocean compared with the reams of penis-shaped graffiti on walls, school lockers and toilet doors the world over, but let's not get all competitive.

It shouldn't really be up to Etsy crafters to educate us on our own anatomy. What we'd like is for there to be more opportunities for women to learn about the clitoris. It starts at school, but it should go beyond. We'd like big YouTubers to talk about it. Can the gaming community share some techniques with each other? Marketing people: how about a Clit-happy advertising campaign for the next cool, ethical brand who asks you to pitch? Let's spread the love.

When we polled our listeners (who are mainly fab, savvy, sassy women and a few fab, savvy, sassy men), most of them couldn't recognise a model of the whole clitoris. There's no shame in not knowing what it actually looks like, but it does show how bad our sex education is. That is because society takes little heed of our wonder organ.

We might think of it as a small pleasure button at the top of our vulva, but this is what the whole thing actually looks like ...

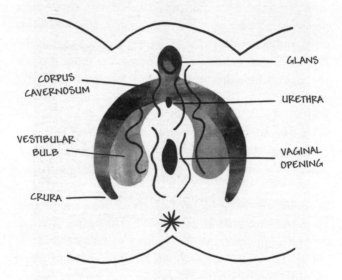

GLANS

CORPUS CAVERNOSUM

URETHRA

VESTIBULAR BULB

VAGINAL OPENING

CRURA

One of our listeners said, 'Is that an abstract painting of me sat with my post-breastfeeding boobs resting on my lap, arms alongside them, wondering what the fuck happened to my body?' She wasn't correct, but it was funny.

Before we tell you some cool things you can do with your clitoris (or someone else's), here are ten amazing facts about this nifty not-so-little organ:

1

The little bead of pleasure located at the top of your vulva, which you may have thought was your clit, is actually just the 'glans'. Think of it like the 'head' of a penis, only more glamorous.

2

The rest of it is made of seventeen other parts, including the 'corpus cavernsum', which are two spongey pillars full of erectile tissue, and the 'crura', which are the 'legs' of the clitoris. The inner lips (or labia) of the vulva are also considered to be part of the clitoris. In total, it can be longer than 10 cm in height. Kind of the same size as a penis ...

3

It is made from the same tissue as the penis shaft and head. When we started out as embryos, we each had something called a 'genital tubercle' which, at the tender age of nine weeks in utero, splits into either a penis or a clitoris. The clit and the penis glans are so similar, in fact, that, biologically, they are considered different versions of the same thing. Think of it as the same clay poured into different shaped moulds, if you like.

4

Such is the disregard science has shown, traditionally, for female sexual satisfaction, the actual shape and size of the clitoris was only discovered in 1998 by an academic called Helen O'Connell at the University of Melbourne. Did you know that spray cheese was invented in 1965?

5

The clitoris contains erectile tissue which, when we're aroused, floods with blood, causing our very own swelling or, if you will, erection. You can find biology-textbook-style photos online of how a vulva looks when the clitoris is erect versus how it looks normally or, for fear of sounding like a 1970s feminist, you can grab a mirror and some lube and have a look yourself.

6

It is often reported that the clitoris contains more than 8,000 nerve endings, which is estimated to be about the same as a penis (some also claim that it has more nerve endings than a penis). Actually, there is no hard evidence for either of these assertions, but we do know that there are a shitload of nerves there, and that women are just as capable of amazing orgasms as men.

Also, the glans on a penis contains the urethra opening too, so in a man it's about piss as well as pleasure, whereas a clit is entirely dedicated to female pleasure.

7

Clitoris is the Greek word for 'key'. Could it be because it unlocks the door to great orgasms? We like to think so. And the bonus is that it's much harder to leave on the bus.

8

Due to its lovely 'spread' across the vulva, the clitoris can be stimulated not just by the skilful application of a finger, tongue or sex toy to the glans, but – depending on how a woman is built – by intercourse, anal sex or frottage/dry-humping genital contact without intercourse. It is thought by some that all female orgasms are a result of clitoral stimulation, albeit from different locations.

9

The plural is clitorises. Just so you know.

10

There probably is a great tenth fact about the clitoris that's worth putting in here. But we haven't discovered it yet. Given its full structure wasn't discovered by Western science until 1998, we think what we do know about it is just the tip of the iceberg (much like the glans of the clitoris), and that our knowledge of why and how this great part of our bodies works will improve to a dazzling degree as time goes on. That is unless there are yet more spray versions of popular dairy products to invest our time inventing instead.

How did reading all that make you feel? Did you know it all? We hope some of you did. We're guessing many of you didn't. It's strange, because we have all been raised into thinking that men and women are different, and that our genitals are the primary marker of this difference. So, to read that, actually, we're not so different after all is a bit head-spin-y. If that's the case, go get yourself a glass of water, possibly a small snack, take a deep breath and come back to us.

So now we know all this, what are we going to do with this knowledge?

Firstly, we hope it gives you some reassurance in the way you experience pleasure. As we talked about in our introduction, most of us don't orgasm through penetrative vaginal sex alone, and is that any wonder, given that most of our sexy nerve endings are not inside the vagina but in the glans of our clitoris?

And although Nineties women's magazines all had us searching madly for a G-spot (supposedly a sensitive area on the anterior wall of the vagina), current thinking is conflicted: while some believe it does exist, and that it's tissue left over from what would have become the prostate gland had we turned into a boy child rather than the girl type, there is also a school of thought that it's all *part of the same thing*, and all kinds of yummy activity, from being licked, fingered, shagged vaginally or up the bottom, using a vibrator, your very own finger, or a delicious combination of any of the above, is hitting a part of the clitoris and the network of nerves which surround it, and getting you aroused ... hopefully to orgasm.

Use this knowledge to educate your kids (male and female). Small children often play with themselves in the bath and are pretty joyful about their bodies. If your four-year-old daughter points to her clitoris and asks you what it is, don't get the bubble bath out and start talking nervously about the picture of Elsa on the front and whether she agrees that *Frozen 2* wasn't quite as brilliant as the first film perhaps? *Explain what it is* (how about 'it's called the clitoris and when you're older it might feel nice if you touch it in private'?). Think back to the 'sex through the tights' chapter and how you want her to be armed with self-knowledge. There is nothing dirty or reprehensible about telling a four-year-old child about their own body. In schools we warn kids about 'stranger danger', but what about understanding their own anatomy?

But moving on from kids ... what about you? We thought it might be convenient to stop here and give you some orgasm techniques because, well, orgasms don't usually just happen to you (unless you get very lucky in your sleep and have a sleep-gasm — this does happen for some). Often, in order to come, you need to relax and clear your mind of thoughts of overdue bills or work meetings or what colour to paint your peeling bedroom wall, you have to focus on the sensations and give your body over to the feeling, squeeze your pelvic muscles or quicken your breath. But, once you know what you like and how to get there, it gets easier and ever more pleasurable and fun.

'I DIDN'T BEGIN ENJOYING SEX UNTIL I STARTED MASTURBATING ... IT'S A SHAME I DIDN'T DISCOVER IT SOONER ...'

Eva Longoria

There will be much more on the subject later on in the book, but for the time being, try one of these.

HOT WAYS TO MAKE YOU HOT

Try a combination of the Hotbed tried-and-tested techniques below and see how they feel. Think of it as a pick'n'mix of pleasure, or a salad of sensation. To help you on your way, pick a lube you like (see the 'LUBE' graphic on p.77), make sure you are home alone (or with a keen partner), that you're not expecting an Amazon delivery and that you haven't left something in the oven. Leave your knickers on to start with if you like (especially if you have a very sensitive clitoris), or take them off and cut to the chase. Dim the lights, draw the blinds, maybe put on a Spotify playlist ... In short, do what you can to make the external environment as relaxing as possible.

- First, try some indirect contact by using your finger to whirl around your clitoral hood, stimulating the periphery of the glans in a windmill-type action.

- Use all the fingers of one hand to pulse the inner labia, as if you were playing the piano.

- Insert one finger ever-so-slightly into your vagina, and just leave it there to put a bit of pressure on the nerve endings here, or circle it slightly, while using your other hand for the other techniques.

- Hold your whole hand out still, and thrust your vulva towards it, experimenting with different speeds and finger positions until you find something that feels good.

- Pull your outer labia out with one hand, and use a finger of the other hand to run around the exposed inner labia, glans and hood.

- Lift and squeeze your pelvic floor (see p.268 for the correct way to do this) and let ago again, on repeat, while you do any of the above, to add an extra internal layer of stimulation.

- Make the 'rawk!' gesture with your hand (thumb and pinkie raised, three middle fingers folded down) and spin at the wrist so your thumb nudges your glans and your little finger touches on your vaginal opening, alternate the pressure between the thumb and the little finger.

- The sex technique app OMGYes! recommends a technique called 'edging', which is nearly bringing yourself to orgasm, stopping, and changing technique until you nearly come to orgasm and stop again, and so on, until you can't take it any more and you have to come. This one is a bit like tantric sex, but without Sting and Trudie Styler.

- Vary the speed at which you do any of the above: try fast then slow, then fast again, until you get into a rhythm you like.

- Similarly, vary the pressure: try a gentle dab-dab-dab around the glans, hood and inner labia, then get firmer and firmer, before going gentle again.

- If you have a free hand, use it to flick or pinch your nipples or, if you're feeling daring, have a little wiggle around or up your bottom — we have a load of nerve endings which help us achieve orgasm, let's use them.

If you like any of these techniques, don't keep them to yourself. Show them to your partner. If they're working on pleasuring you but don't know their way around, don't be afraid to gently take their hand and guide them at a speed and a pressure which you enjoy. There aren't many experiences more excruciating than lying back and thinking about what you can do with the leftover bolognese sauce while a partner is fumbling around, and vice versa. Put them out of their misery! And if you're unsure about how to broach a conversation like this, then try positive reinforcement.

Get louder during the good bits, and quieten down when it's not right. Rather than knock the bits you don't like, scream out what you *do* like about their technique, or praise them for it lavishly at the end, so they do more of that brilliant thing. And if there's something which hurts, tell them immediately. Life's too short for painful sex. Similarly, if you can be a giving and open lover, asking what they like or offering them multiple choice if that's easier ('Do you prefer it hard like this …? Or soft like this …?') then they are likely to follow your example.

While you're at it, you can share the techniques with your friends too. Just as we argued in the previous chapter that a bad sex story shared is a bad sex memory halved, there is no shame in talking about masturbation and, in fact, the more you talk about it, the more it becomes normal, and the better we can all feel. It doesn't need to be a chat that happens at the top of your voices while travelling to work by bus, but during a walk or a dinner or over drinks. We dare you to bring it up: you can say you're reading this book to kick off the conversation … Go.

WHY HOTBED ♡ SEX TOYS

Short of time? Getting a bit bored? It's time to bring in the big guns. Now, let's stop all this nonsense that sex toys can desensitise you. It can be the case that you *get used* to a certain way of coming to orgasm, but you can't desensitise your bits. As part of a varied sex life, there is nothing wrong with a bit of hot pink help (because they are pretty much all hot pink, have you noticed?). Sex toys can make masturbation quicker and easier. One study, by the sex shop Lovehoney, analysed the brain waves of seventeen women while they masturbated with their hands versus a vibrator, and found that excitement levels were actually higher when using a sex toy.

Sex toys are also great to use in partnered sex, particularly if you don't orgasm from intercourse alone. Don't feel as if you're not allowed to enter the toy shop. There is no shame in using sex toys. Many of the best queens and goddesses do.

WHICH SEX TOY? A GUIDE

If you have listened to our podcast, you will know that we get a bit overwhelmed with new-gen sex toys: the ones which come with their own app which you have to install to your phone, and which let someone else con-trol it from their house/abroad. So, we asked the fifty per cent of our listeners who use a sex toy during masturbation, and twenty-seven per cent who use one during sex, to tell us what they use, and here's a guide — in no particular order — to their top five favourites, and ours too:

CLIT-SUCKERS

These tend to look more like epilators than sex toys so could probably pass unnoticed by your mother-in-law if you left it out on the dressing table. They have a tiny opening which you place over the clitoral glans and let the sucking/vibrating party begin!

RAMPANT RABBITS

A favourite ever since it got a mention on *Sex and the City*: these combine vaginal and clitoral stimulation for extra va-va-voom.

BULLETS

Small, quiet and inexpensive, this is a discreet option which works well for women with lots of sensitivity and for using on your clit during intercourse.

THE WAND

This plug-in device, which we think looks a bit like Darth Vader, is like a power tool for your punani, delivering strong vibes and instant orgasms. Not for the faint-hearted.

SPANKERS

These can be quite lovely items that would look very artistic if pinned to the wall in a certain way. The best ones have a leather side for spanking and a soft fur side for stroking. Alternate spanking with stroking for a full range of sensation.

Some stuff to know about sex toys:

- If you are curious at the thought of using a sex toy in partnered sex, but bringing it up makes you want to catch the next train to NeverComingBackVille, try something neutral such as massage oil. This is an entry-level item which can start you on a delicious journey, as, of course, is lube.

- Look for sex toys made from medical-grade silicone as some are made from slightly toxic or porous materials which are not body safe.

- Clean your sex toys after use, ask the shop/supplier for the best method.

- Too embarrassed to go into a sex shop? You can order online and ask for discreet packaging, just in case the neighbour needs to look after it till you get home.

- Know that the ones listed above are a very small selection. You can get strap-on dildos that vibrate, cock rings with fitted vibrators, cock rings that have an added appendage for anal play, toys for trans men and so on. If you suffer from vaginismus you can buy dilators which start small and increase in size. (See Resources at the back for some good people to contact about what is right for you.) And don't forget the lube.

OK, Hotbed, we get it. You love lube. Now can you tell us how to start a conversation with our partner about all this, please?

Yes, we can.

We know how excruciating these conversations can be. We once hosted a live podcast recording in a sex toy shop and, even after that, Anniki only bought a sachet of lube and Lisa bought a wand but left it wrapped up in the corner of the bedroom for two months. It's tricky, we know. If this is you, here are some things that might help:

• Lube up before you start having sex. That way there is no break or awkward moment when you have to say, 'Just chat amongst yourselves for a second while I do something …' Chances are, sex will be ten times better than without it and if your partner comments on this, you can take the chance to say that it's lube and it's from this shop and there's a few other things that might be just as mind-blowing too. It's a good conversation starter.

• Bring it up in the post-sex glow when you're lying in bed, in the dark, looking up at the ceiling.

Did you know that communication is freer and easier when you're not looking at each other directly in the eye? That's why driving and walks and pillow-time are good chances for deep-and-meaningfuls. The post-sex window is a great opportunity to say what you liked about what just happened, and to ask questions that might lead into you making a suggestion that you both love, e.g. 'Have you ever used a sex toy? Would you like the idea of me using a bullet so we can come together?' etc.

- Blame Hotbed! We love blogs and reviews and hearing what you think. Say you're reading a book at the moment, and it suggests using a spanker to get blood flowing to the buttocks, then order one.

- If you really can't bear the idea of talking about sex toys with your partner, or using one together, using them alone for masturbation is still a great way to learn about your body and which areas turn you on. The more you can 'wake up' your vulva, the more you can carry this feeling into your partnered sex too.

THE 'WHICH IS THE BEST LUBE FOR ME?' LOGIC CHART

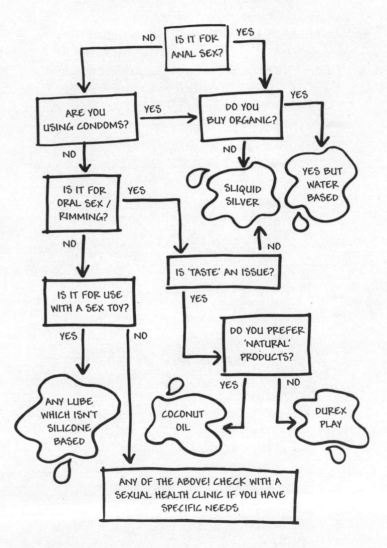

THE HOTBED'S
ODE TO LUBE

(accompanied by a strong beat and deep voice)

Lube, lube, you get it in a tube,

You can put it on your vulva,
and also on your boobs.

It's nice, it's wet and it's shiny,

Certain types are safe for your hiney,

And when you want to be a fast mover,

It can make things that bit smoother.

When your desire is a mere flicker,

It can make things that bit slicker.

Luckily its cost is very low,

Take things fast or take things slow,

Of its praises we love to sing,

Buy it if you can only buy one thing.

WHAT POSITIVE EFFECT DOES HAVING AN ORGASM DURING PARTNERED SEX HAVE ON YOU (PHYSICALLY AND/OR MENTALLY)?

1,185 responses

89.4%

Helps you feel bonded to partner

82.6%

Physical satisfaction

64.4%

Helps you sleep

62.4%

Mental satisfaction

61.7%

Relaxation

58.2%

Increased sex drive / appetite

50.3%

Gives you self-confidence

Other significant answers were 'gives you energy' and 'makes you feel at peace'. In the open-ended section we also got comments such as 'less grumpy' and 'helps with menopause symptoms'.

Orgasms Are a Feminist Issue

4

Flashback to a bathroom in suburban south London in 1986. ANNIKI, aged twelve, and STEPMUM:

> **STEPMUM**
> Please don't shave your legs, darling.

> **ANNIKI**
> Mum, I have to. All the girls laugh when we're doing PE and Angela Rogers called me a gorilla.

> **STEPMUM**
> But why do you need to conform to a masculine definition of female beauty?

ANNIKI
I want one of those Bic razors
like Keeley York has - the one in
a little box with a butterfly
on top.

STEPMUM
I'm not buying something so you
can enter into a lifelong battle
against hair. It's beautiful -
look how blonde it is!

ANNIKI
I'm a big, fat, HAIRY PIG!

ANNIKI
[runs to her bedroom and slams the
door] I'll use Dad's razor. I'll
shave all my hair off. You can't
stop me!

[STEPMUM sighs and puts on a Joan
Armatrading cassette.]

ANNIKI

*The above was a typical pre-teen argument
between me and my feminist stepmum (I
was lucky enough to have a mum and a
stepmum who were feminists). Hair wasn't
the issue. The real issue was I wanted to fit in,
and being hairy wasn't the norm for girls my
age. So, in my tiny teenage brain, that meant
that I couldn't be a feminist either. I wanted a
perm and frosted lipstick.*

The equation was simple.

Feminism = being hairy = people laughing at you in the school shower = becoming a social outcast = hanging out with the class freaks like Wendy Newton who wanted to carry out autopsies when she grew up and smelled a bit.

No feminism for me, thanks!

(Wendy: if you're reading this, I'm sorry and I hope you got the career you wanted and a good deodorant.)

Anniki's stepmum grew her leg hair. She met up once a week with a group of women to discuss radical feminism and how to overthrow the patriarchy. She was pretty damn cool. The problem was, Anniki wanted her stepmum to be someone who was more like Julie Andrews. Someone who baked cookies. Someone who would take her shopping and buy her loads of new clothes. Someone who was fun and not always insisting they go to Greenham Common for their days out (because there was nothing tasty to eat there, it was cold, and there were no boys). Anniki was embarrassed by the books that graced her family bookshelves – Nancy Friday's *My Secret Garden* and *The Joy of Sex*, which she considered a disgusting display of naked hippies.

'I'M A RADICAL FEMINIST, NOT THE FUN KIND.'

Andrea Dworkin

Feminism in the late Eighties, which is now known as second-wave feminism, had rather challenging 'brand imagery'. It wasn't fashionable as it is now. There were no feminist-slogan tees on the catwalk or beautiful men declaring themselves 'he for she'. It required you to reject certain things and accept others. These things weren't compatible with being a popular thirteen-year-old girl.

And it's sad because Anniki, and lots of girls like her, didn't appreciate what changes these killjoy feminists were making for her.

Because, yes, while many women in the Eighties *were* letting their armpit hair grow, this wave of feminism was pretty ground-breaking and positive: they were rejecting traditional gender roles, fighting for equal pay and workplace rights, and becoming more sexually aware. Anniki's stepmum suggested she look at her vulva with a hand-mirror, but this idea felt too frightening and she rejected it.

It's easy to see how a lack of familiarity with your own body can lead to bad sex, right? Let's face it, if you don't know where your clitoris is, then how can you expect anyone else to find it?

What else have these feminists done for us, Hotbed? Discussing feminist ideology isn't the easiest icebreaker on a first date ...

A feminist's work is never done. At least it won't be done in our lifetime. But over the years the feminist movement has helped to effect change which helps to keep us equal, healthy, sexually satisfied and confident. As we have stressed, we are far from achieving these things fully, but these gals have tried their best to at least pave the way so that ...

WOMEN CAN PRACTISE SAFE SEX WITHOUT HAVING TO PUT FRUIT ACID UP THEIR VAGINA

Male scientists can claim a lot of the kudos for inventing various methods of increasingly safe and reliable birth control (before the days of IUDs, the combi-pill and non-latex condoms, women tried all kinds of horrible and ineffective alternatives such as fruit acid, lemons and scalding baths to avoid pregnancy), but feminists have had some influence too. Take for example American suffragettes and friends Margaret Sanger and Katharine McCormick. McCormick funded the development of the contraceptive pill, and Sanger imported the diaphragm to the States from the Netherlands (illegally to start with) and set up New York's only sexual health clinic. The Brits have Marie Stopes to thank for the normalisation and distribution of birth control, although it's worth noting that she was arguably a bit of a racist who did it because she wanted to make sure only middle-class white people procreated ...

WE CAN ENJOY SEX AND ALSO BE SEEN AS A GREAT PARENT AND PROFESSIONAL

Betty Friedan, author of *The Feminine Mystique,* famously pointed out that 'no woman gets an orgasm from shining the kitchen floor'. So-called 'sex-positive' feminists of the Nineties — Kathy Acker and Susie Bright among them — championed the thinking that sex should have no shame for women, that women should enjoy whatever sexual pursuits they were into (as long as they were consensual) without repercussions, and that the virgin/whore dichotomy (the idea that women can either be sexual and shameful, or pure and vulnerable) was total bullshit.

WE CAN BE EQUAL AND BE PRETTY

In *The Female Eunuch,* Germaine Greer argues that women in a consumerist society, obsessed with wealth and nice shiny things, are victims of the patriarchy and taught to hate themselves and deny their sexuality. She encouraged women to break free of the traditional family unit and enjoy shagging around. But she didn't insist that women burn their bras (as some other feminists of the time did), because she saw this as yet another rule from which women needed to liberate themselves. In other words, live as you like, and not as any rules dictate.

WE DON'T NEED TO BE 'CONVENTIONALLY ATTRACTIVE' TO BE ATTRACTIVE

Although it failed to work its empowering magic on teenage Anniki, the pro-body-hair movement of the Seventies was significant in challenging the idea that women all needed to look like Marilyn Monroe (young, hairless, hourglass, white, cis-gendered, able-bodied) to be attractive. Other strands of this thinking, which have flourished in the age of blogs and social media, include the Natural Hair movement, which inspires women of African descent to embrace their natural hair, the Body Positivity movement (see chapter six), and hashtags such as #effyourbeautystandards, #saggyboobsmatter and #GetYourSkinOut. Mexican actress Patricia Reyes Spíndola published a photo of herself in which she revealed her post-cancer surgery breasts under the hashtag #VivaLaReconstruccion, which was bold and dazzling and had a great impact in Latin America.

IF WE DON'T WANT TO BE ATTRACTIVE AT ALL, WE DON'T HAVE TO BE

Susie Orbach's *Fat Is a Feminist Issue* skewered diet culture and described compulsive eating and eating disorders such as anorexia and bulimia as two sides of the same coin, brought about by a consumerist and sexist culture. She claimed that choosing to be fat in a world in which it is not considered beautiful was a powerful feminist statement. Its modern-day equivalents can be seen in the support for Muslim women who choose to wear the traditional hijab or equivalent, and the Sport England campaign #ThisGirlCan which encourages girls and women not to worry about what they look like when they play sport. In her essay and TED talk 'We Should All Be Feminists', writer Chimamanda Ngozi Adichie argues that we don't even need to be likeable if we don't want to be.

PERIODS, PREGNANCY AND THE MENOPAUSE AREN'T GROSS

Germaine Greer urged women to taste their menstrual blood, Patricia Hill Collins wrote positively about motherhood, black motherhood in particular (for example, celebrating the stepmother role, and recognising empowered motherhood as an act of resistance rather than repression), and Gail Sheehy wrote prolifically about the menopause, encouraging women to talk about it, and to demand better provisions for it, such as hormone-replacement therapy.

WE DON'T HAVE TO BE A UNIVERSITY PROFESSOR TO THINK 'FEMINIST'

What's exciting is that feminism is now a movement that everyone can take part in, and many public figures are using their profile to speak out on women's issues. Caitlin Moran's book *How to Be a Woman* made feminist thinking, on topics including periods and porn, clear, funny and relevant to a new generation. The #MeToo movement was started by activist Tarana Burke and galvanised by actresses such as Alyssa Milano, Lupita Nyong'o and Uma Thurman. TV presenter Jameela Jamil campaigns against airbrushing in magazines, calling it a 'crime against women', and she set up the 'I weigh' movement to allow women to reflect on what makes them unique and interesting rather than defining themselves by what they weigh (check out @i_weigh on Instagram). Model Monroe Bergdof has challenged prejudice around transgender identity by posing for

Playboy and appearing on mainstream talk shows as a spokesperson. Angelina Jolie is a UN Goodwill Ambassador with a specific interest in raising awareness about rape as a weapon of war. The list goes on.

It's certainly an *interesting* time to be a woman ('interesting' as in the definition the old Chinese curse suggests, 'may you live in interesting times', i.e. turbulent, conflicted, frightening, disruptive). But let's look on the bright side ...

On the one hand, it feels like we've regressed – women are objectified more than ever, there's still a massive gender pay gap, and there are more men called John leading the UK's biggest companies than women. Theresa May's expensive trousers produce more column inches than her speeches.

There are also a lot of products being sold on the back of 'female empowerment'. Put it this way, there's a lot of ad men banging their fists on the table and shouting, 'Get me some of those feminists on roller skates for my coffee bean campaign!' There's also infighting among the different generations of feminists and social media is shutting debate down: it's easier to sling insults online than to have a proper discussion.

There is still a lot of disharmony between women – a lot of time wasted slagging one another off and criticising one another's decisions and life choices: the way we look, age, date, raise a family, work, communicate, earn a living – the list goes on. As an example, some transgender people are locked in a debate with some radical feminists about things such as whether trans women can comment on 'women's issues' and the definitions of 'sex' and 'gender'. Passions run high on both sides, and sometimes the debate can get in the way of real change.

But change is often painful for many parties. We can't pretend all our feminist ancestors got on like a house on fire (look up 'porn wars' for some context), and we're not all going to agree all the time. Progress is pulling together, realising they are both oppressed groups with more in common than what sets us apart. Some dialogue is happening, and we hope that in five years' time our society will have changed to make sure women and trans people are safe and able to live their lives.

Chill out, Hotbed. Can we talk about sex again, please?

Of course. Taking the conversation back into the bedroom again, isn't it weird that debate has got so far, and yet we still have a long way to go in terms of getting some basics — such as sexual pleasure — right?

Despite being in our fourth wave, despite all the empowering T-shirts and motivational quotes telling women to 'own it' and 'nail it' in their working lives, there are still huge swathes of women who aren't enjoying sex.

It is hard to live a fun, busy life podcasting about sexual pleasure without coming across the ugly old 'patriarchy' word. Try it. What started out for us as a project to put gifs of John Travolta gyrating in his pants on Instagram to cheer up some of our friends, turned rapidly into something approaching radicalism. We know women are sexual creatures. We know hardcore porn can be a bit depressing. We know happiness doesn't lie in spending all your savings on weight loss solutions, and when we start to question it, all paths lead to the patriarchy.

Patriarchy is a system in which men hold key positions of power, wealth and status, and in which men are assumed to be better than women on an intellectual and competence level. In the patriarchy, men (especially, but not exclusively, white, educated, heterosexual, cis-men) are often given the benefit of the doubt, the 'himpathy', and are still sometimes considered a 'top bloke' or 'really game-changing' even in the face of ample evidence to the contrary.

Former US Ambassador Clare Luce Booth distilled it quite neatly when she said,

> *Because I am a woman, I must make unusual efforts to succeed. If I fail, no one will say, 'She doesn't have what it takes.' They will say, 'Women don't have what it takes.'*

The patriarchy has momentous repercussions in the realm of sexuality, and indeed the female orgasm. If this claim seems like a bit of a stretch, read on.

In *The Creation of Patriarchy*, the feminist writer Gerda Lerner outlines her interpretation of how this system of male supremacy is maintained:

> *The system of patriarchy can function only with the cooperation of women. This cooperation is secured by a variety of means: gender indoctrination; educational deprivation; the denial to women of knowledge of their history; the dividing of women, one from another, by defining 'respectability' and 'deviance' according to women's sexual activities; by restraints and outright coercion; by discrimination in access to economic resources and political power; and by awarding class privileges to conforming women.*

It's a weighty list, but one scan of a celebrity magazine or newspaper will serve up any number of examples of women being pitted against one another: on their parenting style, for example, or in a love triangle. Neither is it uncommon to see how many 'rewards' (adoration/fans/followers/jobs/sponsorship deals) a woman gets for being slim, attractive and conforming to stereotypical roles (Marriage! Baby! Weightloss!), and another being ridiculed for being drunk, ambitious or sexual.

The writer Naomi Wolf takes the argument a step further. In *Vagina: A New Autobiography* she argues that a woman who is fulfilled sexually is likely to be more creative, more insightful, more likely to become a business or political leader, and less likely to conform. On a darker note, she asserts that a 'traumatised' vagina is a way of controlling women, which is one explanation of why rape and sexual abuse is used as a weapon of war.

Wolf writes:

> *Female sexual pleasure, rightly understood, is not just about sexuality, or just about pleasure. It serves, also, as a medium of female self-knowledge and hopefulness; female creativity and courage; female focus and initiative; female bliss and transcendence; and as medium of a sensibility that feels very much like freedom. To understand the vagina properly is to realize that it is not only coextensive with the female brain, but is also, essentially, part of the female soul.*

Why are you telling me all this, Hotbed? I thought this book was going to be all about sex toys and lube?

It is about sex toys and lube. It's just that we thought that as well as giving you some practical aspects of the female orgasm, it's also important to add a little cultural, social and political context so that if you do have any feelings of guilt or shame, you can understand some of where they might be coming from (even if you don't have any overt religious or cultural shame around the topic).

Female sexual pleasure itself is, at worst, shamed, silenced, used to sell things or ridiculed, and, at best, seen as a by-product of male sexual pleasure. It is rarely celebrated as something in its own right. There is still a dearth of information about female sexual pleasure, and a lot of difficulty discussing it or showing it.

We live in a culture which is constantly harping on about mindfulness and living for the now, and yet, while experiencing an orgasm is probably the most powerful experience of being *in the moment*, we don't see *any* #ad activity around this.

Many men will say that wanking is a great stress-reliever — in fact, it is so normal we even make jokes about it. We want women to reach that point too, where Sandi Toksvig or Holly Willoughby can joke about masturbation, and for it to be both funny and normal. Caitlin Moran writes about masturbation in her novels aimed at teenage girls, as did Judy Blume, and we want more of this. Remember the scene in *American Pie* where the main character mastur-bates by popping his penis into an apple pie? The cinema edit shows him standing up holding the pie up against him, but in the DVD deleted scenes the character is in fact seen mounting the table and shag-ging the apple pie. It is very funny and it was also ... normal. Boys will be boys. Boys wanking is *normal*. He gets the girl and the happy ending. In both senses.

It's difficult to imagine a box-office smash in which a teenage girl gets herself off in a similar scene. What might that look like? Perhaps she could be testing out the new power shower, when in come a couple of prospective house buyers with their estate agent. Their reaction to her masturbating is one of shock but also acceptance — it's just part and parcel of being a healthy teenage girl, right? Cut to the next scene: the girl is now in a dressing gown, looking slightly embarrassed but also chuffed. Fast-forward to a happy ending in which the girl doesn't get her comeuppance or get chased through a forest by an axe-wielding zombie (isn't it true that in horror films the girl who's in touch with her sexual side is often the first to come a cropper?). Young girls watching our imaginary scenario would leave the cinema with the message that it's perfectly normal and healthy to masturbate and that liking sex doesn't mean that a girl is weird or dirty or that anything bad will happen to her. It's human. Not disgusting or shameful.

We propose a set of new feminist rules. The Hotbed Rules that lead to better sex. We've had a stab at a manifesto but feel free to add your own key objectives.

The thing is, if Anniki hadn't dismissed feminism back in the day, her life would have been very different. Her relationships would have been better. She wouldn't have had so much crap sex. She'd have asked for more.

That argument wasn't about hairy legs. It was all about shaping her future. Happily, she's now catching up.

THE HOTBED FEMINIST ORGASM MANIFESTO

We believe all women …

Have the right to sexual satisfaction

Should be able to enjoy a rich fantasy life if they wish

Should be able to share their tales of good and bad sex without inhibitions and judgement

Should be able to say the word 'masturbate' without going red in the face

Should be able to wear what they want without the threat of sexual harassment or inappropriate comments

Can enjoy porn that is both arousing and feminist

(see chapter on Feminist Porn p.189)

Should ask for what they want including cunnilingus, role-play, anal stimulation, fantasy play – all things more likely to lead to female orgasm

Can choose to be hairy, a bit hairy or completely not hairy

Are allowed to objectify other women and men now and then, especially if these men are Michael Hutchence

(who is unfortunately no longer alive so possibly doesn't mind too much anyway)

Should steer clear of double standards and support one another in the choices we make

Why Sex Education Needs to Go Back to School

5

LISA

My science teacher wore polo necks under skirt suits, and so much taupe eyeshadow it was a wonder she managed to keep her eyes open. I scanned the chapter index of the science textbook for the word 'reproduction', and worked out excitedly how many weeks it would be before that juicy class would come round. That class, surely, would make up for all the osmosis, photosynthesis and Bunsen burner experiments I'd have to sit through in the meantime.

As autumn turned to winter, that blessed day arrived. I nibbled at the end of my Aztec-print pencil and sat there, all ears, waiting for her to begin. 'Good morning, class. Please turn to page eighty-six,' she said as she rearranged the blinds to let in some more weak winter sun. 'Now, I'd like you to read up to page ninety-four in silence,' she continued. 'And, when you're finished, if you have any questions, ask me.'

I couldn't quite believe it. I didn't want to read the pages in silence. I'd already read them in silence at home. Quite a few times. But instead of challenging the situation I did what I was told (funny that this is often the dynamic when it comes to women and sex).

All you could hear for the next twenty minutes was pages turning, chairs shuffling and the classroom clock ticking in the background. Of course, I had questions, tons of them, but I wasn't going to be the first person to ask one. I tugged at my collar, and looked around the room. No one had their hand up. Twenty minutes turned to twenty-five, then thirty. The teacher was doing some marking, and I could hear the sticky ink of her Biro as it ticked and crossed each ruled page. Occasionally she'd look up from under her shiny taupe eyelids, glance around the room for a nanosecond, and get back to her marking.

The bell rang and, as she told us to pack up and go, I'm sure I heard her sigh with relief.

Sex education **SUCKED** in the Eighties and Nineties, when we were at school. There was no mention of the clitoris or how to flick it, no discussion of pleasure, of orgasms. Nothing on how to know you were ready and how to give enthusiastic consent or how to spot it in others. Not a pip on how to recognise if a relationship is abusive or how to help someone experiencing the same.

Neither do we remember any discussion of lube or fore-play; nothing either about boys calling you 'frigid' or making you feel bad for 'blue balling' them, or how you'd feel pressurised to go the whole hog (when actually you liked snogging in their bed and listening to Terence Trent D'Arby, but didn't want more, thank you).

There was nothing about how to stop boys shoving their fingers up your fanny so hard that you winced for a week afterwards. Nothing about booze and sex (or how drinking too much can warp your perceptions and make you fancy people you wouldn't normally). Nothing about how you may not fancy boys at all, but had sexy dreams about Justine Frischmann from Elastica and the older girl who got off the bus two stops before you, instead.

No one warned you that older men might sometimes buy you drinks and that they may not just be kind and friendly and interested in your A-level art coursework theme this spring. (In fact, Anniki knew a much older man when she was fifteen, and wishes in retrospect someone had flagged up that going out to a restaurant, spending time in his bedroom — on the premise of remaking the film *Sleep* by Andy Warhol — and accepting rides late at night **WAS NOT ACCEPTABLE OR COOL IN ANY SHAPE OR FORM.**)

Sex education is all about giving young people the resources they need to make the *right* choices and not end up in bad situations where they're disempowered and on the back foot.

When we hear parents complain about their kids learning about sex at school, we get angry because a kid that is educated knows what to do in certain situations and a kid that doesn't is always going to be in danger of being taken advantage of, right?

In our time, at best, sex education was factual (it was good to know about the menstrual cycle, for example), at worst it was non-existent or tied up with a religious doctrine more intent on upholding a certain morality code than in teaching us the facts. Sometimes it was all of the above. A pupil could learn about the biological act of procreation in a science lesson, something about religion and sin, in RE, and a bit about contraception in their PSHE (Personal, Social, Health and Economics) class, leaving them feeling as if, well, they could have sex, but if they did, they'd probably end up knocked up and burning in hell with a bad case of herpes.

To be fair, some of our teachers may have had the best of intentions, but were not the right people to teach sensitive topics to a class of unruly, hormonal teenagers.

(Lisa remembers another session in which her class was encouraged to put anonymous questions into a box for the teacher to answer. Cue a torrent of piss-take questions such as 'I sat next to a boy on the bus, could I be pregnant?')

Our work on *The Hotbed* is a bit like filling in the gaps on the sex education we picked up in class. It's too late for us to go back to school, but it's not too late to change the record for kids being educated now.

What's depressing is that nothing much has changed since we were schoolgirls. The British curriculum literally has not changed for eighteen years. In 2016, British charity the Terrence Higgins Trust published a report which, after examining the experience of 900 young people aged between sixteen and twenty-five in the UK, found that seventy-five per cent had not been taught anything about consent, ninety-five per cent had not been taught anything about LGBTQIA issues, eighty-nine per cent had not been taught about pleasure, and ninety-seven per cent had not been taught anything about gender identity. Similarly, a report by the UK Youth Parliament, which surveyed 20,000 young people aged between eleven and eighteen in the UK, found that more than half of them had not been told where their nearest sexual health clinic was.

At the time of writing, it is currently only compulsory for British schools to teach the scientific part of sexual reproduction, sex for procreation in other words, and, though we don't doubt that there are some brilliant, inspirational and passionate teachers out there, this teaching can be perfunctory to the point of parody. From September 2020 all schools will be required to teach relationships and sex education – this will include intimate and sexual relationships which is surely a step in the right direction. Parents can take their kids out of class for any discussion beyond the bare biological facts. Also, these rules apply only to council-run schools. Academies and religious schools are not under local authority control, and therefore do not have any obligation to teach anything about sex or relationships. Luckily, there's always hardcore porn, urban myth and clumsy first-hand experiences to help fill this void ...

WHY IT'S NOT ALL BAD NEWS

Thanks to a decision made in 2017 by the Department of Education, the Sex and Relationship Education (SRE) syllabus will be fleshed out and made compulsory in all schools by 2020 (although faith schools will still be entitled to teach it 'in accordance with the tenets of their faith').

How wonderful that sixty years after the invention of the contraceptive pill, twelve years after WHSmith's brought out a range of school stationery featuring the Playboy Bunny logo, and four years after an NSPCC report found that fifty-three per cent of young people aged between eleven and sixteen had accessed hardcore pornography online, schoolchildren will be taught the basics of how it all works by their schoolteachers!

The irony is that rather than encouraging young people to jump into bed with multiple partners the moment the bell rings at the end of their SRE lesson, the more educated young people are about sex and relationships, the longer they actually wait to have sex. A huge UNESCO study of sex education courses around the world found that more than a third led to a delay in sexual activity undertaken by pupils, and a third led to a decrease in the number of their sexual partners.

What is frustrating is that educating people about sex is really quite simple. What young people need is someone to be frank and honest with them, who can explain not only about how reproduction works and how STIs are transmitted, but who can also explain a bit about how our bodies work, how pleasure works, a bit on gender and sexual identity, and the basics on consent and respect, and ... **THAT'S IT**. They don't have to encourage them to go out and have loads of sex, nor demonstrate it with a live show. They don't need to scare kids into thinking that sex is bad or evil, or that sex must only happen within a marriage or purely in order to have children. They just need a bit of common sense and information on real issues that affect them.

In the words of women's rights campaigner and Labour MP Jess Phillips, who we spoke to about sex and relationship education: 'I'm not suggesting we teach children how to masturbate, I'm suggesting we talk to them about the things they're doing anyway.' Having worked for years for Rape Crisis, Phillips believes there is a clear link between poor SRE and abusive relationships: 'To liberate women and end violence is to break down the culture of power imbalance between men and women. Let's stop people feeling ashamed,' she told us.

Doing away with shame chips away at the patriarchy.

Amen.

As we were growing up, we learnt about sex from hearsay. Mainly it was chat about what our friends got up to: being felt up in the corner of a nightclub; one-night stands and holiday romances. In the Nineties we learnt a load from *Sex and the City* when we saw women talk openly about orgasms and oral sex and masturbation for the first time. We saw Charlotte get hooked on her pink Rampant Rabbit vibrator and we bought one too (such is the legacy of this series, the Ann Summers shop now sells one every two minutes).

But then we grew up, settled down, some of us had kids and we started talking about school catchment areas and extensions, and we didn't want our friends to know intimate details about our other halves, especially as, partners in tow, we'd most likely bump into each other at the playground or a weekend barbecue.

And somewhere along the way we stopped talking, and learning. And then we saw statistics around the orgasm gap, and we talked to our friends again, and we talked to our podcast listeners, and we realised that not much sex was happening, and not many orgasms were happening, and that most women couldn't recognise an anatomically correct diagram of a clitoris when we showed it to them.

We are not saying that our poor sex ed classes alone are to blame for this, but we do think good sex starts with good sex education.

Education of women and female empowerment have always gone hand in hand. Education is largely credited with the advancement of gender relations, and the weakening of the patriarchy. It is something to feel strongly about. Malala Yousafzai is a feminist icon, rightly revered for her passionate campaign for education for girls, knowing that to extremists such as the Taliban the most frightening prospect is 'a girl with a book'. Michelle Obama, who has spoken many times about how important her education was to her confidence and her success, has thrown herself into the global campaign for female education. Speaking about the 130 million girls who cannot access even basic schooling, Obama said: 'This breaks my heart, both as a woman whose life was transformed by my education and as the mother of two daughters who wants them and every girl on this planet to fulfil her boundless potential.'

OK, so we are not Michelle Obama or Malala Yousafzai but, in our eyes, a good education is one which includes good sex and relationship education. In our opinion, this is just as important as maths and English.

Women and men, partners, mothers, fathers, grandparents, guardians, educators, podcasters, writers and broadcasters, politicians, health workers — we are all responsible for broadening and continuing the dialogue, for making sure that the right information is out there, to help people learn more about their bodies, their pathways to pleasure, and how to get the most out of their relationships. It's never too late to learn.

TEACHING CONSENT

The #MeToo movement gave voice to stories of sexual abuse in which the issue of consent was considered to be blurred by some critics (otherwise known as gobshites). Some people voiced concerns that consent, or lack thereof, was tricky to define, and tricky to prove. 'Do we need a contract signed now?' cried the sceptics.

During a rape case in Northern Ireland, the lacy knickers worn by the complainant were brandished as 'proof' of her consent and the accused walked free. One journalist wrote about how she was asked to film a consent video before having sex, which is hugely problematic: just because you consent at the time of filming, it doesn't mean you consent if the sex changes key and gets violent, for example, or if you wake up next to each other and you don't want to have sex again. Our favourite description of consent comes from the Rockstar Dinosaur Pirate Princess blog, which was turned into a very cute video (see the link in our Resources section). If you want to teach someone about consent, this is a really good starting point:

'TEA CONSENT'

by Emmeline May
at rockstardinosaurpirateprincess.com

Just imagine, instead of initiating sex, you're making them a cup of tea. You say 'Hey, would you like a cup of tea?' and they go 'OMG fuck yes, I would fucking LOVE a cup of tea! Thank you!' then you know they want a cup of tea. If you say 'Hey, would you like a cup of tea?' and they um and ahh and say, 'I'm not really sure …' then you can make them a cup of tea or not, but be aware that they might not drink it, and if they don't drink it then – this is the important bit – don't make them drink it. You can't blame them for you going to the effort of making the tea on the off-chance they wanted it; you just have to deal with them not drinking it. Just because you made it doesn't mean you are entitled to watch them drink it.

If they say 'No thank you' then don't make them tea. **AT ALL**. Don't make them tea, don't make them drink tea, don't get annoyed at them for not wanting the damn tea.

They just don't want tea, OK?

They might say 'Yes please, that's kind of you' and then when the tea arrives, they actually don't want the tea at all. Sure, that's kind of annoying as you've gone to the effort of making it, but they remain under no obligation, right? They did want tea, now they *don't*. Sometimes people change their mind in the time it takes to boil that kettle, brew the tea and add the milk. And it's OK for people to change their mind, and you are still not entitled to watch them drink it even though you went to the trouble of making it.

If they are unconscious, don't make them tea. Unconscious people don't want tea and can't answer the question 'Do you want tea?' because they are unconscious. OK, maybe they were conscious when you asked them if they wanted tea, and they said yes, but in the time it took you to boil that kettle, brew the tea and add the milk they are now unconscious. You should just put the tea down, make sure the unconscious person is safe, and – this is the important bit – don't make them drink the tea. They said yes then, sure, but unconscious people don't want tea.

If someone said yes to tea, started drinking it, and then passed out before they'd finished it, don't keep on pouring it down their throat. Take the tea away and make sure they are safe. Because unconscious people don't want tea. Trust me on this.

If someone said 'yes' to tea around your house last Saturday, that doesn't mean that they want you to make them tea all the time. They don't want you to come around unexpectedly to their place and make them tea and force them to drink it going **'BUT YOU WANTED TEA LAST WEEK'**, or to wake up to find you pouring tea down their throat going **'BUT YOU WANTED TEA LAST NIGHT'**.

Do you think this is a stupid analogy? And of course you wouldn't force-feed someone tea because they said yes to a cup last week. **OF COURSE** you wouldn't pour tea down the throat of an unconscious person because they said yes to tea five minutes ago when they were conscious. But if you can understand how completely ludicrous it is to force people to have tea when they don't want tea, and you are able to understand when people don't want tea, then how hard is it to understand when it comes to sex?

**WHETHER IT'S TEA OR SEX,
CONSENT IS EVERYTHING.**

The Hot Hotbed Common-sense Sex-Ed Manifesto

When the hallowed year of 2020 arrives, and the reworked SRE syllabus is rolled out, we hope that it will include some of the following principles. And sorry if you are reading this in the future, and we hope the syllabus now looks a bit more like this ...

SEX EDUCATION SHOULD BE MAINLY CO-ED

We are all for dividing up the boys and the girls so they can broach any sensitive topics with a teacher of the same gender, but the facts that are taught should be the same for all pupils. Girls need to know about testicles so they don't knee their mate in the bollocks for a laugh. Boys need to know about periods so that, as boys, they're less grossed out by it, and as men, they can better understand how fertility works and when to fetch their mum/sister/girlfriend a hot water bottle and some paracetamol.

SEX EDUCATION SHOULD BE COLLABORATIVE

Some of the issues raised in sex and relationship education — 'Is it OK to watch hardcore porn?' 'What will my life look like if I'm bisexual and want children?', 'When will I be ready to have sex?' — don't always have simple answers. It shouldn't always be up to a teacher to provide an answer, but instead to offer a framework for critical thinking and discussion, facilitating pupils to come up with their own thoughts around the topics, helped along by solid facts and case studies. It needs to feel inclusive rather than a teacher talking down to a bunch of children who have potentially seen a load of sex online.

SEX EDUCATION SHOULD BE SEX POSITIVE

'Sex positive' is a movement to confirm that all people are entitled to pleasure, whether they be married, single, gender non-binary, cis-gendered, gay, straight, able-bodied or disabled, and so on. Even at school level, everyone should feel part of the conversation.

A connection has been found between the lack of adequate sex education for people with additional needs or physical disabilities and their subsequent vulnerability to being sexually abused. Sex education should encourage young people to understand their body and any changes happening to them during puberty, as well as allowing them to feel entitled to sexual pleasure and in full control of their own body.

SEX EDUCATION SHOULD ENCOURAGE THE USE OF THE CORRECT TERMINOLOGY

As we discuss further later on, the right words are important. When children and young people have the vocabulary to describe what they might be feeling or experiencing in their body, they will be able to express themselves better: whether that be in the doctor's surgery to ask about a burning sensation when they wee, in bed with a partner trying to have an orgasm, or needing to tell someone about being sexually harassed.

We shouldn't be scared of these words: plain, clear words such as vagina, clitoris, penis, testicles, buttocks. They are not dirty or disgusting – they're just part of everyday life (young kids will often revel in these words but then we tend to drum them out of them because we fear what others will think if our kid shouts 'BUM-HOLE!' in a café).

SEX EDUCATION SHOULDN'T BE SCAREMONGERING

Sure, unprotected sex can get you pregnant and give you chlamydia. But with contraception, used correctly, neither has to happen, and sex can be fun and promote deep connection between people. Sex and relationship education should never lose sight of this. And while the teaching can be serious about the facts, it should also allow for a bit of lightness too, because let's not forget that sex can be funny. A fanny fart during intercourse is slapstick humour at its finest and, though it may make you want to flee to the coast to live out the rest of your existence in a cave with nothing but the bats for company, it really is nothing to be embarrassed about. A wet dream when staying at your nan's is the kind of story you should be able to dine out on for years to come. If we acknowledge these moments in class, we're giving young people the tools to be resilient and to know that, if anything embarrassing happens to them, they're not the first person in the world it has happened to. That said, teachers need to make sure they don't ridicule or humiliate pupils, and that pupils are not asked personal questions in the process. One way of doing this is to bring in third-party providers to facilitate the classes: organisations who specialise in this particular area and who can get the tone right.

'"PORN" IS SUCH A BROAD TERM, LIKE PORN CAN BE ANYTHING FROM SOFTCORE AND MELLOW TO HARDCORE, VIOLENT, TORTURE PORN ... FOR SOMEBODY TO LEARN ABOUT SEX FROM PORN I THINK IS REALLY DANGEROUS. AND I THINK THAT HAPPENS A LOT.'

Rashida Jones

SEX EDUCATION SHOULD COVER PORN AND SCREEN SEX

We can't protect young people from porn. No matter what parental controls we put on their phones and iPads, no matter what age restrictions we put on porn sites, or how high up on the shelves we place the jazz mags, there will always be a mate with an unlocked phone, a web company sidestepping the rules or an older brother or cousin with an easily accessible mag-stash under the bed. What we can teach kids, however, is how to understand what is happening in the porn they see. They can be taught that what they may see on screen is designed to shock and entertain, not necessarily to be replicated in real life; about the basic economics of the industry; and that there are alternatives to hardcore porn. (For more on this subject see the chapter on porn later.)

SEX EDUCATION SHOULD COVER RELATIONSHIPS TOO

There is no removing the act of sex from relationships, and therefore good sex education should help pupils understand the difference between a mutually respectful relationship and one which is damaging or unhealthy, and offer them further help with this, if needed. We also think it is important that children are taught that the heterosexual 'nuclear family' – with a mum, a dad and some kids – is just one example of a family structure, and that alternative ways of living (including being single and/or not having children) are options too.

SEX EDUCATION SHOULD BE AGE-APPROPRIATE

Schools need to commit to an ongoing programme of SRE which becomes more expansive as the pupils get older. It is possible to talk to very small children about consent, for example, and how to have ownership over their own bodies, without having to talk about anything too explicit. Likewise, age-appropriate education on porn should start before the average age that a child might see it (in the UK this is estimated to be thirteen).

Recommended Age-appropriate Sex Education Reading and Viewing List

We can't expect schools to take the full burden of our kids' sex education. If you have children, you can encourage open and honest conversations by buying some age-appropriate books or DVDs to read or watch together or to leave out for them to discover in their own time. Make sure you look at them beforehand so you can anticipate any questions.

Here are some books and DVDs we recommend:

MUMMY LAID AN EGG by Babette Cole A very early introduction to sex and conception for younger children, perhaps if they are expecting a new sibling and have questions.

THE A–Z OF GROWING UP, PUBERTY AND SEX by Lesley de Meza and Stephen de Silva Addressing topics such as 'coming out', eating disorders and orgasm, this is an accessible book for teenagers, written with sound medical grounding.

DATING AND SEX: A GUIDE FOR THE 21ST CENTURY TEEN BOY by Andrew P Smiler From consent to contraception, fling this book over to your son and let him know you've read it too.

JASON'S PRIVATE WORLD An educational DVD about a young man with special needs, focusing on topics such as consent.

And not forgetting . . . **MORE ORGASMS PLEASE!** Please give this book to your teenage boy or girl.

GREASE 2

The 'Reproduction' scene in *Grease 2* is exactly what we would have liked our sex ed classes to have looked like: complete with thrusting teenagers, an entirely unflappable, straight-faced teacher, tons of questions (only some of which are piss-takes), and a fab synth-y Eighties soundtrack. Let's forget for a second that the school kids all look as if they're in their early thirties and that Maxwell Caulfield is no John Travolta, and applaud the fact that this scene makes sex seem fun, that questions are encouraged, and that topics such as consent and the menstrual cycle are discussed.

HOW DID YOU LEARN TO HAVE AN ORGASM?

1,199 responses

85.3%
Experimenting alone

43.9%
Experimenting with a partner

15.8%
Porn

11.2%
Magazines

7.2%
Website

7.1%
Advice from friends

6%
TV

4.3%
Films

0.4%
Sex education at school

'Free choice' answers included 'OMG Yes', '50 Shades of Grey', 'the shower head' and 'The Hotbed Collective'. Why thank you.

How Self-Image Affects Sexy Time

6

LISA

Do you want to hear one of the most exhilarating bedroom moments of my early twenties?

It's not about bedding a movie star or getting multiple orgasms on a beach under a full moon. It's much more exciting than that.

I was visiting a friend for her twenty-first birthday at a university in the south-east of England. It was a daytime party in a pub, with games, live music and a lot of cider. So much cider, in fact, that the pub owner had put down straw on the floor to soak up any spillages, be they cider or vomit (I told you this story was going to be exciting).

During one of the games, I started chatting to a very nice-looking guy. He was just my type: geek chic in thick-framed glasses and a trucker cap. Trucker caps were in then (blame Beyoncé) and I was wearing one too. We were doing that quite flirty thing of nicking each other's caps all day, and at the end of the party, although I was meant to be staying with another friend that night, I walked back to this guy's house instead.

After some student-style foreplay (a cup of tea in the kitchen and an episode of The Office *with his seven housemates), we went up to his bedroom. It was here that the trucker caps came off, and so did his glasses.*

'Sorry if I'm a bit clumsy,' he said. 'I can't see much without these on.'

Well, readers, I nearly had an orgasm on the spot. He couldn't see much without his glasses, which meant he couldn't see my body hair, my cellulite, my spare tyre or my small boobs. I was elated.

I flung off my clothes with an abandon never before seen, and was able to concentrate on sensation and skill instead.

We hope by now you're feeling like a part of an educated, open, clitorally clued-up coterie of sex-positive feminists, but even sex-positive feminists can sometimes be struck by body-confidence issues.

Lisa's story is an example of how our fixation on the negatives about ourselves is destructive in many ways, not least as it can really hamper sex and our objectives of gaining orgasm equality. Scientific studies have found that women with a bad sense of body image are less likely to initiate sex, and are more likely to be inhibited during sex, than those with a good sense of body image (it affects men too but to a much lesser degree). And it doesn't matter how conventionally attractive they are, women of all shapes, appearances and states of health and mobility can be affected by low self-esteem.

Why is it that some of us can't separate the joy and pleasure of sex from what we feel we look like when we're doing it?

There is a gigantic difference between [...] me and my Vice-Presidential opponent [...] She's good-looking.
Joe Biden, Vice President of the United States

Never mind Brexit, who won Legs-it?! It wasn't quite stilettos at dawn, but there was a distinctly frosty atmosphere when Theresa May met Nicola Sturgeon yesterday. Daily Mail

Save the whales. Lose the blubber. Go vegetarian.
Peta advertising campaign showing a cartoon of an overweight woman in a bikini.

You do not need to venture far to find examples of women's appearances being commented upon. It often doesn't matter what a woman is doing, whether it be going for a swim at the beach or negotiating Britain's exit from the European Union, but there will be a commentary on her weight, her breasts or her choice of shoes.

It starts young, too. Why is it that little girls are often greeted with comments such as 'Your hair looks so lovely!' and 'What a pretty dress!' instead of 'What are you playing?' or even just 'High five!'? There is nothing inherently wrong with calling a little girl pretty or admiring a woman's shoes. But we think it is important to take a step back sometimes, sip a Martini, and wonder what effect it is having as part of the bigger picture.

Think about what else happens during childhood: before you're old enough to say your own name, you will have been bombarded with gender stereotypes which will inform the way you see yourself. Toys, cartoons and digital games are gendered, with a striking difference between what is aimed at boys and girls. Boys' toys are often associated with strength and action (sport, transport, dinosaurs), and girls' with appearances (princesses, dressing up, hair/make-up). Books are guilty of this too, with a recent study of best-selling children's stories finding that speaking characters were fifty per cent more likely to be male than female.

Before a girl has even started school, she has probably had the importance of her appearance reaffirmed to her time and time again, from many different sources. It's exhausting; not just for girls but for boys too, who can feel pressure to be strong, to 'man up' and not to cry, and to be questioned and sometimes punished for daring to want to wear a princess dress or try on their mother's lipstick. For children with gender dysphoria (when they don't feel as if their gender identity is the same one they were assigned at birth), this must be even more exhausting.

The effects of this obsession with what girls look like are far-reaching, and have an impact on girls long before they have their first sexual encounter. Girls with low body confidence are:

• more likely to develop an eating disorder
• more likely to shy away from socialising
• more likely to skip sporting activities.

We both have very early memories of letting body image get in the way of normal, fun activities:

LISA

My mum is of a strong constitution and didn't often let me or my sister take sick days from school unless we had a leg falling off. One day, however, I was so insistent on feeling unwell, doubling over in 'pain' and pretending to have a headache that she thought, 'What a drama queen', and let me have a duvet day.

The real reason behind my performance? That day I was due on stage in a form play, playing an ant, and I had to wear a leotard. I felt too fat for a leotard, and definitely didn't want to stand up in front of the whole school in one. My only way out of it was to miss the whole thing. I was eight.

ANNIKI

When I was nine, I joined a swimming club. Despite being a pretty great swimmer, I was so self-conscious about my bod that I refused to dive in. It meant I'd have to stand at the edge of the pool with everyone looking at my chubby thighs. Instead, when we did big club races, I'd get into the pool ahead of everyone else and then push off from the side. It drew even more attention to myself because everyone wondered what was wrong. I also developed a way of getting into the pool by shuffling along on my bum. I still do this today. I'm a forty-something woman who shuffles along on her butt rather than stand up in a swimsuit. Sad but true.

THE 'MALE GAZE' IS EVERYWHERE

At The Hotbed, we love a magazine. We love looking at the lovely clothes and the lotions and potions, and reading the celebrity interviews.

But in most mainstream consumer mags, women are depicted uniformly in a one-note fashion: a 2008 study of nearly 2,000 adverts across fifty-eight magazines found that fifty-six per cent of women pictured in women's magazines were depicted as sex objects (judged by criteria such as how their body was posed, what they were wearing and the expression on their face).

In younger women's magazines the figure was a phenomenal sixty-four per cent, surpassed only by men's magazines, where the figure was seventy-six per cent. These women are, more often than not, conventionally attractive — namely white, cis-gendered, slim, young, free of body hair or skin conditions, and able-bodied. A 2017 study by J. Walter Thompson New York and The Geena Davis Institute on Gender in Media found that five times as many women appeared in sexually revealing clothing than men (the same research also found that many more men than women were shown working, speaking and being funny *eyeroll*). And this is before photo-editing kicks in, smoothing skin tone, nipping in waists and zapping away any of those wispy bits of hair around the temples. Is it any wonder that when it comes to sex itself, women can't let go of these sexualised, standardised images and worry about how their body matches up?

NEW MEDIA, NEW PRESSURE

It's all too easy to toke on a spliff and philosophise on a media conspiracy to keep women down.

As Gloria Steinem once said: 'The error that we tend to make is that we think that women's magazines are what editors want and what their readers want — and thus are social indicators — when, in fact, they are what advertisers want.'

While we agree that certain publications perpetuate body ideals and gender stereotypes as a way of pandering to advertisers and to sell copies (sexism sells), it's hard to work out how the conspiracy extends to social media. For every airbrushed, sexualised image in a magazine, there are hundreds of thousands of them whirling around Instagram, which have been doctored by women themselves using easy-to-access and easy-to-use apps such as FaceTune. This is such a new phenomenon that scant research has been done into what effect this is having on people, but some work by the YMCA found that sixty-two per cent of fifteen-to-sixteen-year-olds felt that social media had put pressure on them to look a certain way. More generally, scientists such as those at the Royal College of Psychiatrists are beginning to link social media use with the rise in mental health issues among young people.

'JUST BECAUSE YOU ARE BLIND AND UNABLE TO SEE MY BEAUTY DOESN'T MEAN IT DOES NOT EXIST.'
Margaret Cho

When a social media feed is made up of glamorous selfies and adverts for laxative 'detox' teas and beauty products, it takes some strength of character to think, 'Not for me, I'm happy with how I look!', especially when you are more likely to reel in the 'likes' for a glamorous selfie than the one of you looking a bit rough after a night out on the tiles. It's going to take a lot of work to start unpicking beauty values and how they have been passed on and perpetuated to get to this point, but at least some people are trying ...

The 'body positive' movement is one in which women embrace what they look like, whatever their shape. They post photos or videos of themselves dancing, swimming, doing sun salutations or just having a gay old time. Often, they have soft bellies and plenty of jiggle, and they wear swimsuits and cute dresses and don't apologise for taking up space. The general ethos of the movement can be summed up roughly as the following:

- **All bodies are worthy of respect, whatever their size**
- **You can't judge how healthy someone is from looking at them**
- **Not everyone is meant to be the size society expects**
- **Let's celebrate our bodies for what they can do**

See the Resources section p.347 for some inspiring accounts to follow.

Similar celebratory movements exist for people with skin conditions, body hair, scars or who use wheel-chairs, and we sun-salute them for making it happen. This new vision of the female form, warts and all, is a joy to behold, and following these women is a way of flooding your social media timeline with kickass images that celebrate all kinds of women, rather than just the ones deemed attractive by conventional standards. It does pose its own problems, of course, one of which is that to some extent it still focuses on what women look like, rather than what they can do – sometimes looking at these images we can find ourselves judging and unpicking the women who are being so brave and open with their bodies. This flags up the years of social conditioning that have warped our brains (and how we instinctively apply these rules and negative bias to the women around us) – nevertheless, we think it's a welcome tonic to all the body fascism elsewhere. And, hopefully, the more we expose ourselves to images that disrupt the norm, the more we can expand our tiny minds.

Hey, Hotbed, what the hell has all this got to do with sex?

When you straddle your partner, do you worry about how your stomach looks from that angle? Do you insist on turning off the lights so you don't need to worry about your wiry bikini line? Or never go on top because your breasts flop about and don't look as perky as the ones you see on *Love Island*?

One study describes body-image concerns like these as 'appearance-based distracting thoughts during sexual activity'. Hang-ups about our body have been proven to disrupt sexual satisfaction. In our own research, when we polled people about their sex lives after having kids, we expected the top reason stopping people from having the sex life they wanted to be birth injury or trauma, but what we found instead was that one of the main reasons was poor body image.

In our survey about female sexual pleasure, 'feeling loved/appreciated', 'feeling fancied' and 'feeling body-confident' were joint second most popular answer to the question 'What contributes to you having an orgasm in partnered sex?', second only to 'skill of partner'. Tellingly, only seventeen per cent of people said that 'appearance of partner' was important.

Hey, Hotbed, don't forget that men can feel shit about what they look like too!

Men suffer from poor body image too. This is true. Eating disorders among men are a very real and worrying problem, and men bring their own inadequacies around things such as penis size and premature ejaculation into the bedroom too. There have been calls to stop the 'short dick' jokes from wise people such as our very own Dr Karen Gurney, and Dr Laurie Mintz, who says in her book *Becoming Cliterate*:

> *I was guilty of making such jokes until I realised penis size humour fuels men's anxieties, and these jokes are analogous to men talking about women's bodies in ways that fuel anxieties (e.g. breast size jokes). Ceasing to joke about men's penis size is central to becoming cliterate: if we want men to embrace the fact that their penises are not the key to our pleasure, we need to stop making jokes that indicate that they are.*

From a body confidence point of view, however, men do not suffer to the same degree as women. It is accurate to say that men are not objectified or sexualised as much as women (see p.126 for more on the 'male gaze'), and are therefore less likely to bring distracting negative thoughts into sexual encounters. This could be one more reason why their orgasm rate is much higher than that of women (straight, lesbian and bisexual).

Well, that's something to aim for then, isn't it?

Indeed. In her book *Vagina: A New Autobiography*, Naomi Wolf clearly explains the very interesting concept of the interaction of the autonomic nervous system (ANS) and arousal. There is a lot of medical research into this area, and Wolf distils it nicely. And we will distil it further still.

The ANS is a system your body uses to control some of our unconscious physical impulses such as breathing, shivering and digestion. It is also key to many factors which comprise an orgasm such as heartbeat and blood flow to the vulva — 'the swelling' we referred to previously — which, in turn, creates lubrication and sensitivity. Essentially, in order for the ANS to be fully activated, a woman needs to be completely relaxed. If there is any sense of danger, a woman's responses will be dampened down. It's why, if we're nervous or stressed, it affects our digestion, and why we often don't sleep well in a new environment. Think of 'fight or flight' mode.

In a sexual setting, a woman needs to feel safe in her environment in order to feel aroused. And the safer she feels, the more powerful her sexual response can be. Wolf refers to an MRI study which also showed that the more 'into' the orgasm the woman is, the less inhibited she is in this moment too, the more out-of-body and trance-like the experience becomes. Similarly, research by Harvard University lecturer Dr Justin Lehmiller shows that for women having casual sex, orgasm rates increase with the number of times they hook up with the same person, which tallies with an increased trust as well as an increased knowledge of each other's bodies.

And what about people in relationships? The 'safety' issue struck a chord with us. Because we can feel so vulnerable when we are naked and in bed with someone, there are so many factors which could make us feel unsafe. We're not just referring to standard safety such as not being robbed, or even someone walking in during sex, or finding out that the person we're dating is actually very strange, but also stress factors such as the following:

- That our body will be ridiculed or unappreciated
- That we won't be able to 'perform'
- That we are taking too long to climax
- That we don't feel 'safe' or valued in the coupling
- That sex might hurt due to friction or bad handling
- That our partner might be repelled by our smell or our hygiene.

This tallies with our survey results, which also revealed that low down on the scale of factors contributing to orgasm were those most commonly related to 'sexy' sex, including:

- Risky/unusual location
- Risky/unusual scenario
- Role play/dressing up
- Physical appearance of partner.

When you feel safe, loved and/or appreciated, the more likely you are to be 'in the moment', and the more confident you feel that you are not going to be judged or humiliated while someone is tending to your bits, the more likely you are to come. It's hard to be in the moment when, firstly, you're worrying about the thigh gap, and secondly, worrying about what your partner thinks of the thigh gap.

Again, it is not just those who don't look like a swimsuit model who get thrown off their stroke while worrying about their bodies in the sack. We were interested to read a story about an actual swimsuit model's experience of sex, which you can read in full in *Orgasms and How to Have Them: A Guide for Women* by Jenny Hare:

> *I was a model and I knew my body was stunning. But in a way it detracted from sex as I was so anxious to show it off to its best effect that I spent more time positioning and posturing than letting go and having a good time.*

We think it's sad that instead of leaping head first into a sexual encounter, women so often become a spectator to the act instead — and not a kinky mirrors-on-the-ceiling kind of spectator, but a horrible, bullying spectator, who sits on the bench eating popcorn with her mouth open while pointing and laughing at any tiny body imperfection. Wouldn't it be good if this nasty piece of work could be replaced by a body-positive cheerleader who whooped at our great technique and who cheered when we approached orgasm? A bit like the Teen Angel in the 'Beauty School Dropout' scene from *Grease*, and ideally in tight white trousers and an open-necked shirt, too.

Not all of us will ever have the confidence to share an image of ourselves in our pants on social media.

Equally, we may never go on a nudist beach, do a burlesque dance, twerk in front of a room full of people, or wear hot pants at our fiftieth birthday celebrations, but wouldn't it be good if we at least felt at ease in our own skin when we're doing something fun like having sex?

If body confidence is an issue for you, we would like you to try this exercise. When you are next having sex, for every negative thought you have about your looks, we'd like you to come up with a positive affirmation instead.

This could be a nice thing about your appearance (if you really struggle with this, ask a good friend to help you: we can be so much nicer to each other than we are to ourselves), or something about how the sex makes your body feel rather than what you look like.

Here are some examples of how to move the practice into the bedroom and concentrate on how sex feels rather than what you look like, make you feel like a goddess, and get up the orgasm rate as a result:

NEGATIVE THOUGHT	POSITIVE AFFIRMATION
My boobs are saggy	It feels great when my nipples are pinched
My bum is too big	I love it when I'm kissed along the knicker line
My scars are ugly	This person is in bed with me because of who I am
My stomach isn't flat	The skin on my stomach is soft and sensitive
I haven't waxed my bikini line	My vulva is soft and sensual when it's wet
I need to lose weight	I love how my hips and waist look when I lie on my side
I hate my body	I am great at giving head
I'm not as hot as his/her ex	My skin is a beautiful colour
Why is he/she interested in me?	I'm a great kisser

It's quite trendy these days to pin positive affirmations around the house, so you can remind yourself of what a legend you are as you load the dishwasher. We'll add Sex-Positive Mantra Cards to our long wish-list of 'Unusual Hotbed Merchandise' but, in the meantime, just write your own list of nice things to say about yourself and every time something negative pops into your head, tell it to get lost and bring in the big guns instead.

OTHER WAYS TO FEEL BODY-CONFIDENT IN BED

MINDFULNESS TECHNIQUES: You know those mindful meditation techniques which implore you to focus on every little flavour of your mouthful of food, or to acknowledge your negative feelings before sending them away? These all help you to get in the relaxed mindset for good sex, or 'mindsex', if you like. Focus on the orgasm and not on what you look like. Think about your breathing, squeeze and release your pelvic floor, tweak your own nipples, concentrate on each sensation, notice how your partner's skin feels, think about every move the two of you are making and how they feel. It's quite similar to the process of getting to sleep, in this way, i.e. anxiety makes it hard to fall asleep, but focusing on your breath as you inhale or exhale, or squeezing and releasing muscles, or noticing how the sheets feel against your skin can all help you get off (to sleep).

CURATE YOUR MEDIA: Unfollow people who make you feel shit, follow the body-positive movement, or equivalent, to remind yourself that all bodies are worthy of love and sexual pleasure. Watch some diverse women having sex on Make Love Not Porn rather than mainstream porn. Stop watching TV shows that use body-shaming for jokes if this gets you down. Remind yourself of the male gaze (see p.126) when you are watching films, TV or porn.

EXERCISE: Not to alter your body shape, but to give you energy and boost endorphins, which both help with body image and sex drive.

WEAR SEXY BUT COMFY PANTS AND UNDER-WEAR: We're not getting bossy here, but scratchy, too-tight underwear or a soiled T-shirt with a cartoon of Snoopy declaring **'I HATE MONDAYS'** might not make you feel as sexy as some underwear that you treated yourself to and makes you feel a million dollars. This is not about conforming to the patriarchy but is more about wearing things that don't make you feel like *a human wet wipe with zero sass.*

COMMUNICATION: If low body confidence is affecting your sex drive, talk about it with your partner. Chances are that they will reassure you that you are a goddess and a queen, and — if you have been avoiding sex for this reason — they may feel relieved to find out why and realise that they can help tackle the problem: whether that be changing how they talk to you in bed or discussing any underlying issues. If they can't reassure you and/or if they say anything which undermines you further, then that may be a red flag for getting further help with your relationship.

THERAPY: If past trauma such as sexual assault or bullying is affecting your body confidence or making you feel unsafe in the bedroom, there is specific therapy which can help you. See the Resources section for more information.

CHANGE THE SETTING: Soft lighting, a warm room (even socks if you can bear it) and clean sheets can help you get in the moment and feel comfortable and safe. Think Kate Bush video.

HAVE SEX AND MASTURBATE: It's a bit chicken and egg, but sexual satisfaction can actually help to boost self-esteem.

REMEMBER YOU DON'T NEED TO 'PERFORM': Screen sex will make you believe that you have to fling yourself around the room naked, or dress up as Catwoman. While both these things are great if you have the whim, great sex can still happen under a duvet in the dark.

GET INVOLVED IN A FANTASY: Close your eyes and think of something sexy. This can either be alone or shared with your partner. Fantasy can focus the mind away from undermining thoughts and onto the physical sensations. No ideas on where to start? Read on to the next chapter …

WHICH OF THE FACTORS BELOW CONTRIBUTE TO YOU HAVING AN ORGASM DURING PARTNERED SEX?

1,191 responses

78.8%
Skill of partner

66.5%
Feeling fancied

65.2%
Feeling loved/appreciated

64.7%
Feeling body confident

43.5%
Feeling clean

27.5%
Fantasy (in your head)

24.1%
Sex toy use

22.9%
Physical appearance of partner

---

*We asked the same question about masturbation and the top three answers were 'Fantasy (in your head)', 'Sex toy use' and 'Porn/erotica'.

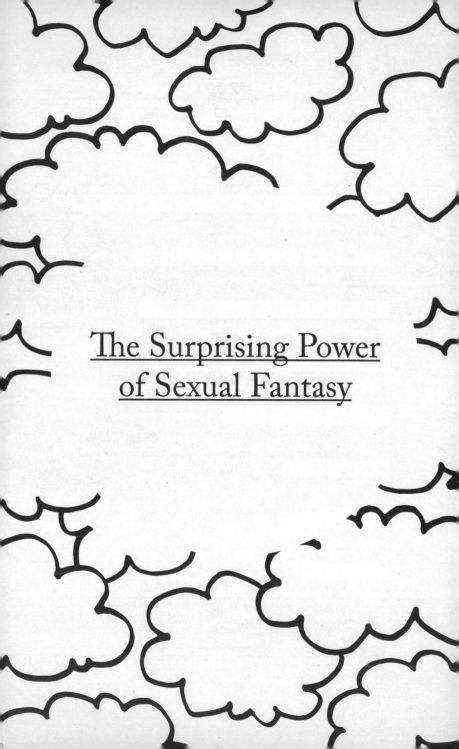

The Surprising Power
of Sexual Fantasy

7

ANNIKI

Simon Le Bon has one arm wrapped around my shoulder and is whispering into my ear. 'I've never met anyone quite like you,' he says seductively.

I smile sheepishly. I am out shopping wearing a frumpy, floor-length nightie and can't seem to find my way home again to get dressed.

'You're the most beautiful girl I've ever seen,' he says.

We wander around the shop arm in arm. There are second-hand books for sale, retro furniture, and food stalls serving snails and French cheese. Simon keeps me close and every time I move away, he pulls me back.

'You're so refreshing because you're nothing like Yasmin,' he says.

'That's true, I guess,' I say, trying not to feel offended.

Simon doesn't know that I changed my second name to Yasmin when I was twelve because I wanted to be more like his gorgeous supermodel wife.

'Shall we find somewhere more private? Wouldn't that be fun?' he says, smiling cheekily.

He has those silver-grey highlights that were extremely popular in the mid-Eighties. He is wearing a linen boiler suit that I've possibly seen a style influencer wear on Instagram.

'I just need to get out of this nightie and text my partner,' I say.

I worry that Paul will be wondering where I am. I also feel guilty that I like the idea of finding somewhere more private (once I've sampled a delicious triangle of brie, perhaps).

When I wake up the bedroom is boiling hot. I'm embracing a pillow. Simon has evaporated without even a puff of smoke. I shut my eyes

— trying to welcome him back so we can find somewhere more private. But he's gone.

I am bereft.

At The Hotbed, we're obsessed with fantasy, day-dreams and night dreams, how they interact with physical pleasure and what they might mean. Our imagination costs nothing and can reward us so richly, and yet we're often discouraged from letting it run free. It's time to change that.

When you were a teenager you probably enjoyed a rich fantasy life, and if you could have looked inside the brains of your female friends you would have discovered that they were dreaming just like you were. Sometimes these fantasies would have involved celebrities, and might have been pretty banal (watching videos with Corey Feldman, in Lisa's case or foxy sex on a spaceship with John Taylor, in Anniki's case).

For many young people, fantasy is the only regular sexual experience they have, and allows them to prepare themselves emotionally and physically for forthcoming encounters in real life. In our pre-teens and teens, we go through puberty and those first few sparks of sexual attraction start cropping up. The supply teacher who makes us blush, or more commonly the pop star or actor we are obsessed with. We lie in our beds with our floral duvet covers, thinking about what it would be like if we hung out with these men or women in real life.

What would we talk about?

How would they touch us?

Where would we want them to touch us?

What would we do together?

Eventually we go on to have real sex. We perhaps conform to certain expectations. As we've outlined in previous chapters, we don't prioritise our own pleasure, because we haven't been educated about our own bodies or how to orgasm, or we feel negative about the way we look. We worry that our tummy wobbles too much and our boobs are different sizes. All these things get in the way.

What's great about the fantasy world is *anything* is possible. If you want to sit on George Clooney's face while staring out at the Aegean Sea – get to it. Perhaps you are on tour with Beyoncé and she invites you backstage for some extra dance practice. Or you find yourself in the plot of *Killing Eve*, sandwiched between Eve and Villanelle and there's only one way you're going to be allowed out of the room alive. How about a double date with Michael Fassbender and Idris Elba, where they get into a fight over you on a busy Soho street, and then one or both of them take you out dancing (or maybe you head straight to the hotel)?

Fantasies aren't just for teens. They're valuable, what-ever stage of life you're in. It's important not to let boring, humdrum adult life take over. It's sometimes useful to access that side of yourself that dreamt about sex before you knew what it was like.

If you're a new mum and feeling tired, emotional and overwhelmed, fantasising about someone you loved in your twenties may help you feel more normal and alive again. If you're in your forties and feeling bad about ageing, maybe you fixate on a rock god.

Why else should we give ourselves permission to have a fantasy life? Because it's exciting. There's a sense of expectation. The unknown. It allows us to love and be sexual without having to deal with rejection (fantasy partners are usually totally into us). So, we know we can forget about any body hang-ups or physical barriers (e.g. living with your parents, a physical disability, illness) which might hamper the real thing.

What's not to love?

And remember that ANS thing we mentioned earlier? It's the system your body uses to control some of your most unconscious impulses like breathing and digestion. In order for the ANS to get busy and do what it should, a woman needs to feel relaxed. In fact, the safer she feels, the more powerful her sexual response is likely to be. And fantasising about people we don't know, or used to know, or would like to know, is relaxing, right? So, more fantasising equals easier activation of the ANS. Fantasy also allows us to explore dangerous and transgressive scenarios but in an ultimately safe way.

We may have belittled teenage girls because they had crushes on Justin Bieber or taken the mickey out of the woman on the tube reading *Fifty Shades of Grey* (there was certainly a lot of patronising push-back against the book, which was dubbed 'housewife porn' or 'mummy porn', when it first came out), but instead we should view these as practical tools that help women relax, feel safe and more readily tap into what turns them on.

Fantasy is one of those things that plays a pivotal role in shaping our sexual identities. Whether it's a more passive dream-state like the one Anniki describes, or a fantasy that we actively construct ourselves, these imaginings help us to understand what really turn us on.

All too often women are taught to believe that a male construct of sex is the most arousing. Giant penises. Frenetic penetrative sex as seen in porn. Women fainting because they've caught sight of a big willy and orgasming before they've removed their bras. The nice thing about fantasy is that it lives in our heads. It rebels. It does as it damn pleases. It can truly represent our desires.

Hey, Hotbed, stop daydreaming and give us some science!

Fantasy has a physical function too. A study by the University of Louvain in 2014 found that women who have 'erotic thoughts' during intercourse were more likely to have regular orgasms than those who don't.

Similarly, a study in 2011 which surveyed 3,000 Australian female twins found a correlation between women who climaxed during masturbation with those who could think wild-and-sexy during sex. In our listener survey, thirty per cent told us they use a fantasy to help them orgasm during partnered sex, and ten per cent share a fantasy with their partner. Fifty-two per cent use it to come while masturbating.

Let's say that again: if you fantasise you are more likely to have an orgasm.

WHAT CAN WE LEARN FROM NANCY FRIDAY?

So, what are women thinking about while they orgasm? For the real juice, we strongly recommend that you read Nancy Friday's book *My Secret Garden: Women's Sexual Fantasies*. It's nothing short of mind-blowing.

Nancy Friday asked hundreds of women to share their sexual fantasies with her. Under the safety blanket of complete anonymity, these women revealed fantasies that were as wild and as daring as you can imagine. Many of them are beyond our own imagination, which makes them even more enjoyable and mind-opening to read.

My Secret Garden was groundbreaking at the time because it revealed that *yes*, women fantasised and that oftentimes these fantasies were transgressive and wild (one of the fantasies involved a woman who dreamt about having sex with an octopus in another, a neighbour's dog gets involved). They talk about these sexy stories starting on autoplay in their heads the moment they start to get excited. Before Friday's book, it was assumed that women thought about baking and nice ironed slacks while they masturbated, if they masturbated at all. Friday's book made talking about fantasy more permissible, and revealed how rich and exciting that dream state can be. It's also very normalising, because whatever your sexual fantasies are, it's likely there is something just as taboo and out-there in the book.

Interestingly, Friday's work was derided for not being academic or scientific enough. She sold millions of copies.

So, Hotbed, what are the most common female fantasies?

A study in the *Journal of Sexual Medicine* (in which 1,516 men and women were interviewed) revealed that sex in unusual or 'romantic' places were among the most common female fantasies. 'Taking part in oral sex' and 'performing oral sex' were also in the top five, with seventy-eight per cent of respondents saying oral sex was top of their fantasy list. 'Being masturbated by a partner' followed closely behind. We have to take these findings with a pinch of salt as, like most studies, it is limited by various factors. In this case, a big problem with the data is that the fantasies were written out as survey questions, which the respondents then checked if they agreed. This check-box exercise is no match for a woman's wild and fierce imagination.

The results are still interesting, nevertheless. According to this study, the ultimate fantasy for many women would be a scenario where her partner performed cunnilingus and stimulated her clitoris. It's not exactly tentacle sex. Neither is it something we see in mainstream porn very often, and yet reflects the fact that most women won't climax without clitoral stimulation. Indeed, fantasies can potentially reveal an absence, a need that is currently untapped.

My Secret Garden was published almost half a century ago. Many of the women interviewed were housewives: many got married young and had only known one or two sexual partners. Their fantasies, therefore, are perhaps a reflection of not having the same experiences many women can now boast about: many talked of strict upbringings and puritanical parents, and admitted that this guilt gave them an added sexual thrill. Similarly, Friday isn't the only person to opine that because women's desires have so often been suppressed, their fantasies frequently contain an element of being dominated or forced to do something sexually daring or extreme. In fantasising in this way, the women were exploring their sexuality without carrying the guilt of taking part in the act.

Friday did a couple of follow-up books, including *Women on Top* in 1991, which featured more women-on-women and women-in-charge fantasies, which she said reflected the inroads to equality made by women in the preceding decade. The fantasies were so wild that the book was banned from several libraries in the US.

We live in yet more permissive times, and although we haven't found true equality with men yet, we have more options than ever before. At the same time, with careers, children, daily exercise, nightly meditation, monthly detoxes, quarterly declutters and all the other things we are told we need for a full and happy life, there are simply not enough hours in the day to devote time to sex and masturbation. So, are our fantasies different as a result?

'IN MY SEX FANTASY, NOBODY EVER LOVES ME FOR MY MIND'
Nora Ephron

We asked our listeners to send in a description of one of their fantasies. We didn't make it a 'tick-box' exercise so they could run wild. Common themes were sex with people they weren't supposed to have sex with (e.g. a partner's friend, therapist or senior colleague), sex with other women (even if they define themselves as straight), group sex, and being watched, encouraged to orgasm or dominated. Here are some of the fuller responses we received:

I sometimes fantasise about my husband masturbating and me watching without him realising I'm watching (like peeking through the bathroom door when he is in the shower or coming home from work and he is in bed and doesn't know I've come home).

I'm having sex with a man, usually I'm on top, but I'm being watched by others (mainly men) and they're all massively turned on by me and what I'm doing and how sexually aroused I am. And sometimes a second man joins in ...

I am a heterosexual cis-woman, but most of my fantasies involve me being a man and having sex with women. I have no idea why. But I like to think of myself as having a huge, insatiable penis, having to bed woman after woman until I come to my own climax.

FANTASIES AREN'T NECESSARILY REFLECTIVE OF WHAT WE WANT TO HAPPEN IN REAL LIFE ...

It's important to remind ourselves that just because the thought of something makes us horny ... it doesn't mean we *want* to do it in real life. Fantasies provide a 'safe space' where we can let our thoughts run wild without causing any physical hurt or upset to ourselves or others.

Women often fantasise about being dominated, tied up and even raped. Indeed, a 2009 study of 355 college women at a north Texas university revealed that sixty-two per cent of women had had such fantasies. These kinds of fantasies can make women feel ashamed – why am I thinking about this awful stuff? How can I be a feminist and enjoy rape fantasies? Is it really OK to think about being tied down and raped while I'm masturbating?

If you join in the #MeToo campaign, march to 'reclaim the night', take part in a #SlutWalk and call to boycott any film or drama which has a gratuitous, sensationalised rape scene, is it also justifiable to defend any woman's right to fantasise about being violated? Why does it happening in a woman's head suddenly make it OK?

Well, if it comes up at drinks parties, this is what we say: rape is a crime, a horrible crime, and one which has a shamefully low conviction rate. Anything in real life which encourages victim-blaming or which normalises the crime is dangerous. Lastly, anything which uses rape to make money (films, porn) and may sometimes be painful to perform, is a world away from what might happen in a woman's head, which doesn't hurt anyone, doesn't encourage it happening in real life, and has no impact on anyone other than on her. It's a tough one, but we got there. Canapé, anyone?

No thanks, Hotbed. I'm off home ...
What was the best way to try out a fantasy?
Asking for a friend.

There are several things we can do to make the most of our fantasy lives:

- We can stop feeling guilty and realise that fantasies are normal and fun — even if we believe them to be strange or have no interest in acting them out in real life.

- If you can't think of your own sexual fantasy, read *My Secret Garden*. One of the fantasies is bound to turn you on.

- Remember that fantasies can provide a vital means of escape, helping us to re-access parts of ourselves we've put to one side or simply to bring some magic back into the routine.

- Should we choose to, we can use fantasies to help fuel our sex lives. So, telling your partner about the things that turn you on can help them better understand what makes you tick, sex-wise, and can be a hot activity in itself. Just be tactful and don't tell them if you want to give their brother a blow job. And also, remember not to laugh at or belittle their fantasies

- Try exploring your fantasy along with a sex toy and/ or some lube. Vary different types of touch while you fantasise. Lick your lips, stretch out your legs. Mix it up, treat yourself.

• Finally, playing out your fantasy in your mind can be a useful mindfulness technique. It doesn't cost anything. It can help us zone out of our everyday lives and focus on the sensation of the love-making or masturbation.

So, whatever it is that turns you on, be it watching your partner having sex with a stranger or eating cheese with Simon le Bon … don't feel bad.

Close your eyes. Enjoy it. Revel in the fantastical.

IS THERE A FANTASY (FANTASIES) WHICH HELP(S) YOU REACH ORGASM?

1,185 responses

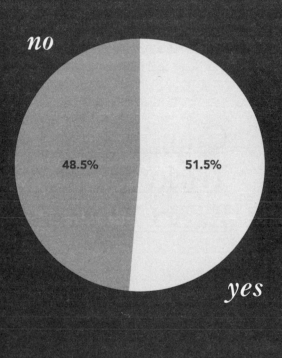

no

48.5%

51.5%

yes

338 people also described their most effective fantasy to us. These included 'being worshipped by multiple men', 'lesbian fantasies although I'm confident I'm hetero', 'situations I've been in with a partner', 'someone watching me have sex' and more.

Cunnilingus: Tricky Word, Easy Orgasm

8

ANNIKI

When I was in my teens, nobody talked about cunnilingus.

Boys.

Blow jobs.

Yes.

But cunnlingus?

No. Nada. Nothing. Natch.

On the rare occasion that it did come up, it was often accompanied by a wrinkled-up nose and more than a smidgeon of disgust. This was no doubt linked to the shame we felt about that part of our anatomy. We thought our nether regions were a bit peculiar and weren't surprised that the opposite sex had the same thoughts too.

Blow jobs were the name of the game. If a girl wanted to be popular then the onus was to learn how to perform them, refine her technique, and in return she could expect a pat on the back (and, as word tended to get around, being asked out by lots of boys).

The more I think about those days, the ANGRIER I feel. The fact that cunnilingus was ignored meant that it didn't get onto my list of sexual expectations. It wasn't normalised. Subsequently, I had adult relationships where it didn't happen and I didn't think that was weird (perhaps I thought it was something rarefied and special and only happened two or three times in your life).

Then later when it happened, I felt awkward because I wasn't equipped to ask for what I wanted or to relax and enjoy it.

Instead I felt like I needed to go and buy the guy in question a present because he'd undertaken such a heinous, disgusting, unrewarding task (when he was simply giving me the self same pleasure I'd given him).

I came to the conclusion that cunnilingus just wasn't getting the airplay it deserved.

This idea that we need to feel *grateful* to anyone who gives oral sex is absurd and one we need to dispatch right away. However, it's a belief that exists. Or there's a sense of embarrassment and general ickiness surrounding it. And yet, when done well, it can be *the best thing in the entire universe*. In fact, even when not done very well, we think it's still one of the best things in the entire universe. Let's face it, there probably aren't many women lying on their deathbeds, secretly wishing they'd had *less* cunnilingus.

Cunnilingus is high pleasure, low effort for women and, if more women had oral sex, it would certainly help close the orgasm gap: oral sex is one of the reasons attributed to why the orgasm gap is smaller for lesbians. It's not rocket science — lesbians tend to enjoy more oral sex.

So, why aren't we all more into it? We think it's probably to do with the fact that society doesn't place a priority on female pleasure or fully acknowledge that it involves the clitoris, and, as we've discussed before, the clitoris is still a mysterious body part for some people; that, yes, you might not quite know what to do with when you get down there. Cunnilingus remains intimidating because of this lack of information and may be an 'out of bounds' area for teenagers.

The embarrassed silence around the topic begins early on at school, then those awkward feelings and shame often follow us into adult life.

For women sleeping with men, there are more barriers and fears associated with oral sex than for women sleeping with other women. We'd like to see more cheerleading of this lovely act: let's get the showbiz reporters to stop asking celebs when they're going to have another baby, and to ask them to say something nice about cunnilingus instead. If you are an Instagram influencer, why not use the #blessed hashtag for next time you get great head? TV scriptwriters, more oral sex on screen please! It's a part of a great sex life, it's free and it's normal.

To focus for a moment on men specifically, because women who a) have sex with women and b) don't do oral sex are, from our understanding, few and far between, we found it interesting to note that some of the most pivotal, groundbreaking cultural figures of the male variety — men who've created great art, music, literature, film — are men *who do go there*.

TAKE THE ARTIST FORMERLY KNOWN AS PRINCE. Prince DID cunnilingus. In fact, he sang all about it on his infamous album *Dirty*. The song 'Head' includes the lines, 'I'll give you head till you're burning up. Head till your love is red.'

This was a man who wasn't scared of pleasuring women. A man who practised what he preached. He was also a genius.

WHAT DO YOU THINK TO DAVID BOWIE? Another influential and pivotal figure in music history, and here was a man who also performed cunnilingus – in fact, Bowie simulated the act of oral sex on Mick Ronson's guitar in public, on stage during his Ziggy Stardust heyday.

DWAYNE JOHNSON, THE ROCK: WE LOVE YOU. When the musician DJ Khaled told the host on *The Breakfast Club* radio show that he never went down on his wife because 'It's different rules for men ... We the king. There's some things ya'll might not want to do ... it got to get done. I just can't do what you want me to do', the Rock responded by tweeting: 'Ahem ... *clears throat* as a man, I take great pride in mastering ALL performances ...'

MICHAEL HUTCHENCE (Anniki's favourite pin-up) – well, of course he enjoyed cunnilingus. We're sure of it. *Look at the man! He is also a genius* (if you're not keen on INXS's later work, try their first couple of albums – *Shabooh Shabooh* and *The Swing* – you may be pleasantly surprised).

Going further back through history, you have those famous literary darlings of the Bloomsbury set. We're sure they did it all the time. Geniuses all.

AND WILLIAM SHAKESPEARE? Well, we're guessing here, but we think he probably liked a bit of cunnilingus after a hard night sweating over his latest masterpiece.

(Please note that we haven't conducted a scientific study into the correlation between 'being good at oral sex' and 'creative-genius-like status', but if there are any big institutions who would like to gather robust data around this theme, we'd be interested to hear if our theory is true.)

Men who are comfortable doing cunnilingus tend to be men who are happy in their own skins, men who prioritise pleasure for their partners, men who aren't childish about tasting their partner, aren't scared of getting it wrong, want to see their lady having fun in the sack and above all they don't behave like a bunch of silly five-year-olds who've spotted a dog poo in the park and squeal and run away.

It would be good to think that expectations among young people are changing from the days that Anniki went to school. Sadly, this doesn't seem to be the case. In 2016 researchers Ruth Lewis and Cicely Martin conducted a study for the *Journal of Sex Research*. Lewis and Martin interviewed boys aged between sixteen and eighteen, and discovered (depressingly) that while, in theory, these boys believed male and female pleasure to be equivalent, in practice they saw performing oral sex on a girl as a 'bigger deal' than receiving it, i.e. a girl giving a boy a blow job. *Vice* magazine reported on the study stating: 'The prevailing idea among the teen boys that vulvas were "dirty", "disgusting", "nasty", "droopy" [...] "messy" [...] and "stinking". That meant, therefore, that oral sex on women was undesirable work.'

In short, the boys' opinion was that giving head to girls was dirty, not high-status, and therefore not worth the effort. *eyeroll*

When you twin this kind of attitude with exposure to porn and how vulvas are now expected to look a particular way (hairless, the inner labia ideally concealed or removed entirely) then you can see that the prejudices towards cunnilingus have probably become worse (and for women there's more shame about what their vulva looks like rather than less). The desire for the vulva to look a certain way, to smell a certain way, to conform to certain criteria only makes cunnilingus more awkward and less likely to happen (it's very hard for a woman to relax and activate the ANS if her brain is cluttered with all these concerns).

Why aren't men schooled more in cunnilingus? Let's have a look at popular culture and see whether that's helping to prioritise cunnilingus in any way, shape or form.

The notorious 1972 film *Deep Throat* stars Linda Lovelace as a woman who discovers that her clitoris is in her throat, so to achieve orgasm, she must give men blow jobs — ideally taking the penis as far back into her throat as possible.

Depressingly, when we look at modern porn, women are still depicted gaining pleasure and achieving orgasm through 'deep throating' men. Is this because some of the 'scriptwriters' in the porn industry still believe that this is where the clitoris is located?

CAN WE JUST SPELL IT OUT? THE CLITORIS IS NOT IN THE THROAT. AND AS FAR AS WE KNOW, ONLY A VERY SMALL MINORITY OF WOMEN WILL ORGASM BY GIVING MEN BLOW JOBS. (If you are one of these women then please get in touch as we'd love to hear more about this experience.)

It doesn't help that Sigmund Freud, still hugely influential in how we see and understand the world of sex and relationships, was pretty down on clitoral orgasms. He saw them as the annoying little sister of the voluptuous, sophisticated vaginal orgasm, and taught that women who were unable to orgasm vaginally were sexually immature. No, *you* are!

To right this wrong, seeing as porn and popular culture celebrate blow jobs and the women who give them, what about a film that we might call *The Champion Diver*? Has anyone made a film about a male character who gives oral sex to women and this is the entire narrative of the film? And what if men orgasmed ONLY through giving cunnilingus? Would this change the sexual dynamics somewhat? (We're sure that oral sex for women wouldn't need a drastic rebrand if this was the situation – it's a shame really, even if the film would be a little same-y.)

Accepted, in some cinema there might be a romantic vision of cunnilingus, a vision where the man dives under the duvet, and the woman experiences orgasm before he's unhooked her bra. This kind of myth doesn't help. Oral sex is a skill. In the same way that giving blow jobs is a skill. There's technique, and there are things to avoid (more on this later).

Thankfully, there have been a few signs recently that popular culture is catching up with how cool cunnilingus is. For a start, we are occasionally seeing it on TV. We are also seeing oral sex in a more believable light, i.e. not something that gives a woman an orgasm before her partner has even reached her pelvic area. These are encouraging signs, but we need to see more of this kind of realistic and honest sex in popular culture and on our screens: sex scenes in which women are on the receiving end of oral sex rather than the obedient providers. If we believe that women deserve more orgasms, if we want to close the gap, then this is clearly one way forward.

COMMON CUNNILINGUS CONCERNS AND HOW TO CONQUER THEM

I THINK I SMELL WEIRD

These fears are often founded in our adolescence and the references people made to the way women smell 'down there'. You may have heard boys talk about girls being fishy, musky, sour, vinegary ... the list goes on. The sad thing is that men often don't suffer with the self same smelly labels when it comes to their penises (when in reality there are a variety of odours and not all of them are pleasant).

The main way to conquer this fear is to wash your vulva. Just with water. Nothing with loads of synthetic fragrances in (these are likely to make you itchy and uncomfortable). Shower. And smell yourself. The thing is, the vulva has a natural smell and every woman is different. Chances are your partner will like the way you smell (or maybe you have the wrong partner rather than the wrong smell?). If you are paranoid about how you taste, would it be so awful to taste your own lady-juices? A teensy droplet on a fingertip will do it. You will realise that it often doesn't taste of much. Maybe a bit salty. Sometimes sweet. It's not really a big deal. If your vulva's smell, taste or discharge changes then just take yourself to your local sexual health (GUM) clinic (or GP) if you are worried. Many causes of this kind of thing are temporary and can be treated.

I MAKE A FUNNY NOISE

Yes, this really can be an issue. The sound of someone lapping at your clitoris can make a bit of getting used to. We women are not used to making rude noises — and these noises are definitely *rude*.

Get over this by listening to music. Prince might be a bit too heavy-handed in the bedroom but maybe some old-school Massive Attack?

If you really want to be CLEAR on your expectations, how about:

'Go downtown and eat it like a vulcha.'
'Work It' by Missy Elliot

'Put your dirty angel face / Between my legs.'
'Twist' by Goldfrapp

'What are you afraid of?'
'A Taste' by Bikini Kill

'I don't want dick tonight / Eat my pussy right.'
'Not Tonight' by Lil' Kim

I FEEL VULNERABLE AND EXPOSED

It's true that oral sex is possibly one of the most intimate things you can do with another person. As women we're taught to sit with our legs crossed, be ladylike, prioritise others. Cunnilingus is the opposite of that. It requires placing yourself at the centre of the universe, lying back, relaxing in a way that doesn't come easy. It requires accessing a part of yourself that is so relaxed that you're almost asleep but in a nice way. It requires turning off the list-making, rational, worrying side of your brain and pretending you're lying on a deserted beach, your out-of-office is on, and the suncream is applied.

There's no easy way to get over this. Try closing your eyes and focusing on your breath. Try not thinking about how the world is going to hell in a handbasket.

And if you still find that you're not up for it, you're not up for it. That's fine too.

WILL I FART?

This can be a legitimate concern, and yes, it happens. When your body relaxes then it's only natural. Who cares? It's not the end of the world. You just relaxed your muscles. Big deal.

Think 'What would Madonna do in this situation?' Chances are she'd make light of it, chuckle and then get back to business. She wouldn't roll off the bed and run to the bathroom crying. Madonna wouldn't cower in shame.

I HAD A BAD EXPERIENCE AND CAN'T FACE IT

We've got a whole chapter on bad sex, and cunnilingus is one of those things that, when it goes wrong, it can scar you. Maybe your partner was too enthusiastic. Maybe too rough. Maybe they stuck their nose in your vulva thinking it was sexy and tried to nose-fuck you. Maybe they kept looking at you with a moustache of your own pubic hair, and brought up something about your mother. Maybe it's all those things.

Like riding a bicycle, get back on. Use the classic 'shit sandwich' technique (which works for every delicate conversation, from feeding back in an appraisal through to optimising cunnilingus skills). Say something like, 'I loved it when you did X but wasn't so sure when you did Y. Can you do more X in the future?'

I WILL MAKE A WET PATCH

Yes, you might. Good sex can mean a variety of fluids: spit, lube, spunk ending up on the sheets. And isn't that brilliant? Wet sex is good sex, so consider your wet patch a badge of honour, like a Blue Peter badge with focus on the 'blue'. Sheets can be washed.

Sometimes we turn into people who are tidying up mess before it even happens. Don't be that person. That person doesn't usually get much pleasure out of life.

So, there you go. As you have probably gathered, we're big fans of cunnilingus. Unfortunately, though, a bit like snogging, it tends to go out the window in the long-term relationship. It becomes a distant memory like laughing at one another's jokes, sharing puddings and playing footsie under the table in restaurants.

BUT IT DOESN'T HAVE TO BE THE END. See if you can reintroduce it into your life. Be more demanding. Remind your other half that it's a path to creativity, genius and true talent. Flatter. Quote Prince lyrics.

Do what you must to get your end away.

GET AHEAD AT GIVING GIRL HEAD

First up

Try it and stop putting it off for a special occasion. The time is now.

Second up

Go gently. The clitoris is very sensitive and different women respond to different levels of pressure. This may be direct or less direct. Start off with a soft motion and then you can build up the intensity.

Third up

Look at your partner and see how they're responding. If they're gritting their teeth and doing a similar face to when they gave birth then ease off, change your technique. If she's flopped out like a Persian rug, licking her lips, and moaning or panting, if her legs are shaking, she's probably enjoying it. It's a bit like kissing. Go with your gut but you can also ask her the kind of yes/no questions that you might get from someone washing your hair at a salon: 'Is this slow enough?' 'Is this a good pressure?' and let her know she can say no and you won't be offended.

Fourth up

Try a circular motion with your tongue but also a horizontal movement that goes back and forth across the clitoris.

Fifth up

We know this is hard, but if you have the energy/appendages, try inserting a finger or two into the vagina as your partner becomes more excited, flick a nipple, lightly rim her anus (making sure anything that touches her anus does not then touch her vulva — bacteria, man).

Sixth up

When she's close to orgasm, try the technique called 'edging' where you ease off for a bit, take your mouth away and then go back a few seconds later.

Seventh up

Don't expect to be bought dinner/a new jumper/not to have to take out the recycling for a week as a reward. Also, don't immediately request oral sex or a blow job in return. In an ideal world, let your partner relax and enjoy the post-orgasm calm. Feel smug that you are someone who **DOES CUNNILINGUS** (and wait for our scientific study to be published which will hopefully prove that geniuses do and numpties don't).

Everything You Want to Know about Bum Sex but Were too British to Ask

9

LISA

Sal* was a friend of a friend at university. She was fun, confident and clever. She had a boyfriend in our fresher's year. He talked her into having anal sex and, even though she wasn't really into the idea, she said yes to please him.

The experience was awful, far worse than she'd imagined it would be. It hurt and she bled. Bad enough in itself, but worse was when she got a text message from him the next day. 'Did anal with Sal last night,' it read. 'Fucked her right up. It was amazing.' That mis-sent text message, and the proof of fuck-wittery within it, got him promptly dumped like a load of toxic waste and she got on with her life.

*Name changed and story told with her kind permission.

I, on the other hand, was so horrified by her experience that I was never able to even entertain the idea of bum sex. Too painful, too high-stakes.

THIS BUM SHOP IS SHUT!

Get away from that area. You have no business here.

Jog on.

Oh, the bum sex. That's one conversation starter. So much to say. And yet you can't really bring it up at Sunday dinner, or while you're queuing outside your spin class. It's a shame, because there are so many myths to bust, so many complex feelings to unpack, and so much joy to be had.

Of all the topics we broach in this book, anal sex is probably the one which is the most tied up with guilt, shame and misunderstanding. We considered writing a whole book on the topic, but fear of what our parents would say (and what we might put on the cover) held us back, and this kind of tells you all you need to know.

And if we told you we were all fighting over writing the intro to this chapter, we'd be lying. It's still one of those subjects that makes women cringe.

Fessing up to being a big anal sex fan creates a real sense of vulnerability. What will people say? What will they think? What if I'm the only one who actually likes it? And yet, what a coincidence that, when we put out a podcast about anal sex, entitled 'I'd Like Something Up My Bottom, Please', it was one of our most-listened-to episodes.

Here are some myths about anal sex which may have put you off:

- Anal sex is dirty
- Anal sex is for gay and bisexual men only
- Women can't enjoy anal sex
- Being a woman who has anal sex makes you subservient
- You can't be a feminist and have anal sex
- Painful anal sex should make you scream with pleasure like a porn star.

Hey, Hotbed, stop saying 'anal sex'!

We can't! We're saying it lots of times to normalise it! Anal sex. Anal sex. **ANAL SEX**.

Now, please give us a moment while we clear away the bullshit. *fetches a spade the size of a continent and shovels away the shit*

Hey, Hotbed, is that a reference to the fact that some people might equate bum sex and 'tossing the salad', as the cool kids call rimming, with actual poo?

It wasn't actually, but now we're on the topic, we should mention anal play and hygiene.

Yes, the anus is where the poo comes out but, in between bowel movements, very little, if any, remains in the anus or rectum. You can have a little wash before partaking in bottom play, and even wear latex gloves for fingering the anus, if that's your vibe. Both partners should also wash their hands in between touching a bumhole and a vagina, just to avoid any bacteria being transferred from one to other. If you know anal play is on the sex menu, how about putting a flannel by the bed/floor/sex swing for convenience, or making sure one hand is for bum and the other is for vulva? Different condoms and/or sex toys should also be used if you're going from anal penetration to vaginal.

The lining of the anus is thin and easily damaged, therefore anal sex is riskier than other forms of shagging, and a condom should be worn for any penetration unless you've both just been tested for STIs. There's also a risk of urinary tract infections for both the 'top' and the 'bottom'. But … we wouldn't be realistic if we didn't acknowledge that, in relationships in which you're both sure you are free from anything contagious and neither one of you is having unprotected sex with other people, this may seem a little over-cautious.

If you take these precautions, anal sex and anal play do not need to be dirty or disgusting at all. And if it's your thing, it's totally worth the extra faff.

'HE TOSS MY SALAD LIKE HIS NAME ROMAINE / AND WHEN WE DONE, I'LL MAKE 'EM BUY ME BALMAIN.'

Nicki Minaj

'IN THE UK, WE HAVE THIS THING WITH BUMS'

We have a funny relationship with our bums in the UK. We've grown up on a diet of *Carry On* films, which were full of references to farts, bums and poo. We see builders' cracks and can't help but snigger. We feel uncomfortable thinking about bums and poo and all that stuff in the same breath as sexy, yummy, lovely things like orgasms. We've built a culture of titillation and Frankie Howerd-style jokes around bottoms, many of which have a homophobic twang to them. Let's nip this in the butt.

Which moves us neatly on to the next prejudice.

'ANAL SEX IS ONLY FOR GAY AND BISEXUAL MEN'

(Actually *pushes glasses back up nose*) ... Recent surveys of sexual behaviour show that many lesbians lurve anal sex too. There doesn't need to be a penis in play for anal play to be part of the game. A strap-on dildo will do quite nicely, thank you. Or a tongue. Or a finger. Anal action is on the rise for straight men and women too: a 2009 survey published in the *Journal of Sexual Research* showed that one-third of heterosexual women had tried anal sex, compared with one-fifth just ten years before. But what is also interesting about the survey is that only ten per cent of heterosexual women reported having anal sex in the previous year, which shows either that the ones who tried it didn't like it (horses for courses), that they didn't know how to get the most pleasure out of it, or just that they see it as 'event' sex and not something to be incorporated into their regular or semi-regular shenanigans.

'WOMEN CAN'T ENJOY ANAL SEX'

This myth probably derives in part from the fact that for men, anal play can stimulate the prostate gland, which can give them a rather wonderful orgasm, but as women do not have a prostate, it cannot. However, men and women have an equal number of nerve endings in their bottoms, meaning that it can be as hot for a woman as for a man. Not only that, but some of these nerves are linked up to the clitoris, so anal stimulation can help you achieve a clitoral orgasm. Depending on how a woman's body is built, the anal sex or anal play can also stimulate the vagina or the clitoral legs. In other words, ring-a-ding-a-doo-dah!

'BEING A WOMAN WHO HAS ANAL SEX MAKES YOU SUBSERVIENT'

With so much focus on men's pleasure, it can be true that certain sex acts make you queasy. If there's nothing in it for you, why should you take part? Especially when there's something really good on TV. We hear ya, sister, and we don't judge. And if you are in a relationship or a hook-up in which you feel pressured to do bum stuff when you don't want to, then this isn't a healthy place to be (see Resources at the end if you need help getting out).

However, if you are curious to try anal sex and want to know what it feels like, please know that your bottom is just another area of your body, and should hold no more guilt or shame than your little finger or your earlobe.

'YOU CAN'T BE A FEMINIST AND HAVE ANAL SEX'

Well, it depends what kind of feminist you are. Andrea Dworkin famously wrote a book called *Intercourse*, in which she asserted that all male-to-female intercourse in a patriarchal society is so degrading it is akin to rape.

If you adhere to Andrea's school of thought, then no, perhaps you shouldn't have anal sex. But we're in the fourth wave of feminism, and thankfully, we believe that a woman's body is her own. Your body, your choice.

So, it's fine to have anal sex if you enjoy it, and to not have anal sex if you don't. Choices, y'all.

'PAINFUL ANAL SEX SHOULD MAKE YOU SCREAM WITH PLEASURE LIKE A PORN STAR'

Eep, no. No, and — once again with feeling — **NO**. Anal sex should not be painful, full stop. And if it is, please stop, full stop. Porn sex can be hot to watch, but as we will discuss further in the following chapter, it isn't realistic, and probably shouldn't be used as a how-to guide. For tips on non-painful, sexy bottom sex, read on ...

HOTBED'S HANDY, CUT-OUT-AND-KEEP ANAL SEX FACTSHEET

1

Women have a load of zingy nerve endings in their bottom.

2

The clitoris can also be stimulated via the back passage.

3

While the anal tissue is prone to tearing due to lack of natural lubricant, if practised properly, anal sex does not need to be painful.

4

And while the anus is also for pooing, if you take correct steps, anal sex does not need to be dirty or disgusting.

5

If a man wants to try anal play, it does not have to mean that he is gay.

6

Anal sex does not always mean a penis in an anus, it can also include using a sex toy, a dildo, a strap-on, or using your hands or mouth.

7

Women can enjoy anal play as part of their sexual vocabulary.

8

There is no shame in liking anal play, whatever gender or sexuality you are.

9

There is no shame either in NOT liking anal play.

THE HOTBED GUIDE TO
SEXY ANAL SEX

In the 2017 study of heterosexual women's views on anal sex published in the *Journal of Sex Research*, it was also found that while some women had tried anal sex out of curiosity and enjoyed it, many were also put off by the fear of pain, and shame. But why is it that many logical, sensitive women have so much fear of having something in or around their bottoms? Is it porn and its apparent obsession with harder, faster, longer anal sex? Perhaps you tried it and didn't like it? Or is it simply because the general silence about anal sex means we don't know enough about it and how to make sure it is pleasurable for both parties?

If you've read all the above and the thought of anal sex or even any anal play is still absolutely not your cup of tea, then move on to the next chapter. It is your body and your choice, and there is no shame in deciding that it isn't for you. Shut your shop, tell people to jog on. But, if you are tempted to explore how it might feel, here is our guide to getting to the bottom of it.

1. Unlike the vagina, the anus is not naturally lubricated, no matter how turned on you are, so please use lube for any anal play. But remember that many lubes are not compatible with condoms, so look for water-based rather than oil-based lubes, the latter of which erode condoms.

2. The safest place to start the Great Bottom Experiment is on your own in a safe and quiet place such as your bedroom. With a lubed-up, clean finger (preferably one which doesn't have a long, bejazzled nail), have a little tickle around and just inside your bumhole. You can try this while masturbating or using a sex toy on your clitoris, and you can even try it first with your pants on if this makes you feel more relaxed.

3. If you wish, have a good wash before you start. Run tepid shower water over your bum crack and use your hand to have a little scrub. If you want to go industrial, you can douche the area with a special shower head attachment, which restricts the waterflow and which is easier to clean. You can buy these from any mainstream plumbing store. Or you can get a bulb-shaped anal douche from a sex shop. Fill with lukewarm water and gently squeeze into your bottom while sitting on the toilet. Gently expelling the water will also expel any extra poo into the toilet. Repeat until the water runs clear. Be aware that some research points to an increased risk of infection after douching.

4. The most sensitive areas of a woman's anus are near the entrance, and on the front wall of the anal passage (because this is where it backs on to the vagina). Don't forget that the butt cheeks are highly erogenous too, so there's plenty of mileage for fun with your buttocks.

5. Rimming is when one person licks or sucks another's anus. Heaven for some, hell for others. If you would

like to try it, incorporate it into a body massage, where you kiss and tickle the super-sensitive butt cheeks as well as the butt hole.

6. If your sexual partnership doesn't involve a cis-male with penis, you can still have bum fun with rimming, fingers or sex toys. 'Pegging' is the practice of anal sex using a strap-on penis or dildo, and the same rules for lube apply. You could even try this as a woman in a heterosexual relationship with a man. Anything goes.

7. A word on butt toys and the like – these are becoming increasingly popular and can provide an easy entry point (no pun intended) to anal sex. The important thing to point out here is that anal sex toys need to have a wide base to avoid them being pulled up inside you, so please don't use your standard toys for backdoor fun.

8. Finally, an extra top tip (for tops?) from sex educator Alix Fox: when you are partaking in any kind of anal play, do not use a lubricant which contains numbing agents. Some lubes are designed to make anal sex more comfortable and might contain a small amount of anaesthetic such as benzocaine but, if you can't feel the signals your body is sending to tell you that you're not ready yet, that you're not stretched and dilated enough for someone to put a toy or a penis in you, or if there's a small tear or an abrasion, there's much more chance that you will do yourself damage. Anal sex done slowly and properly shouldn't hurt. If it does, it could be a sign that you're taking it a bit too fast or that something has gone a bit wrong.

So, there you go ... we hope we've made the concept of anal sex less frightening. We hope we've demystified it a bit.

And remember you're cool if you do it and you're equally cool if you don't. No judgement here.

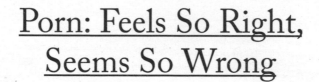

Porn: Feels So Right, Seems So Wrong

10

ANNIKI

Last year I decided to embark on a bit of a social experiment. I decided to watch porn every day for a week. Let me also tell you that … I've never …

- *Squirted*
- *Been penetrated by a dildo that is as big as a tree trunk*
- *Been penetrated by two/three men at the same time*
- *Dressed up as a schoolgirl*
- *Had lots of men come on my face*
- *Peed on someone or been peed upon*
- *Been in a gang-bang (though I once snogged three men in one night back in the Nineties).*

Perhaps my existence has been sheltered, but day one of my 'grand porno experiment' and I notice all these things are de rigueur in your average porno. I see very little that resembles my own sex experience (am I too vanilla in my tastes? Too boring?). I also notice that none of the women have any hair on their vulvas. And that the sex is often rough. Like make-up-streaming-down-the-face-because-I'm-crying-a-lot rough.

It's disturbing. There is zero foreplay too.

On day two and three, I notice that all the men are obsessed with penetrating things. This might be a vagina or a bum or a wall or a doll or an envelope. The style is often what I'd describe as 'Jack Russell on heat' — fast, and relentless. Nobody got the memo that slow and sure can also win the race. I start to feel a bit guilty that I'm aroused by some of the clips (like I've done something bad; that the woman is definitely faking her pleasure for the camera), then worried that I'm too judgemental and perhaps she does enjoy it, but how can we tell?

I watch a woman having multiple orgasms with a dildo the size of a Dyson vacuum. From her pained expression I worry that perhaps 'more orgasms' aren't always a good thing?

Day four and five and I'm struck by how sore the vulvas look and how they'd benefit from a good, calming soak in warm water, or a nice cooling compress.

I'm also alarmed that messages keep popping up on my screen asking if I want 'a rough, old MILF to fuck who lives locally'. Have I accidentally offered my services by clicking on the wrong banner?

Day six and seven and I'm jaded. I'm seeing balls, penises, tits, arses and sore bums everywhere. When I see a local dad in the park, I immediately picture two women standing on either side servicing him. I end up staring at two dogs in the park as they get it on, and miss my daughter pleading for an ice cream as the van drives away. I feel more guilt.

The porn is definitely impacting on my visual repertoire. I am also feeling like I want to watch more (and wondering whether dogs getting it on are arousing or is it just my pornified mindset?).

Pretty depressing really ...

Your attitude in public to porn probably depends on what circles you move in. In some worlds, admitting that you watch porn is a bit like saying you pick your nose or wee in the shower: it's a bit gross and shameful, but you're not the only person who does it. In other circles — usually in a 'men's locker room' scenario or around younger people — admitting that you *don't* like porn is a bit like saying that you worship God (i.e. it makes the other person feel immediately as if you are judging them).

'I THINK PORN, LIKE ANYTHING ELSE, CAN BE ENJOYED. IT CAN BE PRODUCTIVE FOR BOTH MEN AND WOMEN.'

Scarlett Johansson

We think it's OK to admit that you are confused about porn. We are. Many of our listeners are. As feminists, watching porn raises some tricky issues.

We did an episode called 'Can Feminist Porn Give You the Horn?' in our first-ever series of *The Hotbed*. We each watched a load of feminist porn to work out whether porn without a lot of the hallmark features could give you the panty-thumps as much as the standard stuff (more on that later). We were flooded with messages from women who said it was the first time they'd heard women talk openly about watching porn. Many women said they watched it but felt guilty about it. Others loved it unashamedly. Hardly any of our listeners had heard of feminist porn or, as we want to call it, 'ethical porn' (because 'feminist porn' sounds too much as if Andrea Dworkin had hooked up with Angela Davies and got hold of a webcam).

Heterosexual porn is a conundrum to us and here are some of the reasons why:

PROS

- It can be a shortcut to feeling aroused
- It can be fun and entertaining
- In some cases it can be healing/therapeutic
- It's easy to access
- Being judgey about how others are turned on isn't cool
- It is legal (well, most stuff)
- It's popular
- Some women make a lot of money through porn
- It is a huge industry which employs lots of people (not just the actors)
- Many of the people in the industry enjoy their jobs
- It's as old as time.

CONS

- It can perpetuate a very narrow view of female beauty (slim, young, large breasts, pouty mouth, small and symmetrical inner labia)
- It can perpetuate myths around male sexuality (e.g. that big penises are superior to smaller ones)

- It often perpetuates white supremacy (i.e. white porn stars make the most money and people of colour are often fetishised, e.g. 'Asian babes')
- It often depicts degrading acts towards women
- It often fixates on penetration and places other activities on the back burner
- It sometimes depicts degrading acts towards men
- It rarely depicts genuine female pleasure
- Men make more money out of the industry than women
- The outfits/hair/settings are usually terrible.

But Hotbed, surely anything which gives us a shortcut to pleasure is a good thing?

Well, yes. To an extent. But it's a tricky one because while it can be arousing, it's hard for us to keep the 'Cons' out of our mind when we watch it.

As data journalist Mona Chalabi says in her *Guardian* video series 'The Vagina Dispatches': 'I think there's always this question when you're watching porn of like, "Are you really having a good time right now, though?"' It confuses us to get our rocks off to something as loaded with potential ethical problems as porn. In other words, our body likes it but our brain doesn't.

Let's elaborate on some of the Pros and Cons.

THE CLOTHES/HAIR/SETTING ARE TERRIBLE

This isn't just a joke, it's a real thing. We watch porn and we think, 'What a horrible shirt!', 'That flooring looks too cold to have sex on', or 'Those kitchen units have seen better days'.

Also, the men all seem to be from some Eighties body-building gym. Where are the Paul Smith suits? The interesting facial hair? The sexy banter?

Porn directors of the world, times have moved on.

A couple of scientific studies have found that the details *do* actually matter more to women than men when watching porn. One study used eye-movement trackers to find out where men and women were looking and, although both sexes looked at the actors' bodies, it found that while men looked more at the faces of the women on screen, the women taking part in the survey looked more at the surroundings. In another study, men and women were asked why they found various different porn films arousing: more men than women rated the sexual attractiveness of the woman as key to what turned them on, while women tended to be turned on if they felt they could see themselves in the scenario. So, if that scenario involves a bathroom that looks as if there might still be skid marks down the toilet, then the women would be less lightly to get the horn. But give us porn set in flats with the kind of furniture you'd find in *Elle Decoration* and undies which are more Agent Provocateur and less lacey-and-scratchy, and we would enjoy it more.

IT CAN PERPETUATE A VERY NARROW VIEW
OF FEMALE BEAUTY

Pornland author Gail Dines, a slightly unpopular figure in 'sex-positive' and 'pro-porn' circles due to her dogged critique of the medium's current state, refers to 'F**kability v Invisibility' in her TEDx talk 'Growing Up in a Pornified Culture'. She thinks the pornographic male gaze has infiltrated our culture to the point where it is grooming young women to think they must be sexualised and sexually available to be 'seen'. The male gaze is, as we discussed in chapter 6, a bit of a fucker.

And the pornographic male gaze, which favours one type of feminine beauty above others, could be the reason why labiaplasty (the surgical alteration of the inner or outer labia) is becoming quite eye-wateringly popular. Although the numbers are still relatively small, it is now the world's fastest-growing cosmetic procedure, and the women who are requesting it are increasingly young, which makes us want to cross our legs protectively as we write. The most common reason for having labiaplasty is not to do with pain or sexual pleasure (although some women do have the op for these reasons) but simply to alter the appearance of their vulvas, with researchers pointing to porn and the media (social media, television and magazines) as an explanation. Vulvas are as different to each other as our noses, eyes and knees, but if the only vulvas we see are the standardised porno model, we might start to think we're not normal. We will stand up for the right of adult women to alter themselves in any way they choose, but should we stand by and let the porn and cosmetic surgery industries influence how we feel about diverse bodies? We think not. Especially, as we have discovered, as the inner labia contain part of the clitoris and therefore should be held sacred. Not trimmed and chopped ...

CONFIDENCE → SHAME FLOW CHART

STEP ONE: Make women feel not beautiful/sexy/clever/good enough
↓
STEP TWO: Allow a solution to fix the 'problem', which costs women money
↓
STEP THREE: Make women feel guilty for choosing to 'fix' the problem
↓
STEP FOUR: Create another reason for women to feel not beautiful/sexy /clever/good enough

repeat to fade

IS PORN ADDICTIVE?

Well, isn't this the big question? It's a good question because it hasn't really been answered yet. Porn 'addiction' is not listed as an actual disorder because there is no hard evidence to show it is. In fact, some studies suggest that many people who seek help claiming they are addicted to porn just believe they are because of the feelings of guilt or shame they have around watching it. It can also be a bit chicken-and-egg: has my relationship broken down because I'm watching porn, or am I watching porn because my relationship is breaking down? and so on.

But there are people who think their relationship with porn is problematic. Paula Hall describes herself as a porn addiction therapist, and she runs a clinic for 'sex addiction', including compulsive porn use, In her TEDx talk 'We Need to Talk About Sex Addiction', she said:

> *Since the advent of the internet and smart-phones anyone can get hooked. Easy access and no education on risk means that more and more people are getting addicted without even knowing that it's happening.*

She compares the fast and private access to porn now with pre-internet times when you couldn't 'turn the pages of a *Playboy* fast enough' to get hooked.

It is also believed that the body and brain can start to crave a stronger hit, or at least something different, each time to get the same result, just as they do when it comes to other stimuli such as food. Some people talk of needing to watch more extreme, more degrading films. An academic study in 2018, which looked at the interplay between gender, race and aggression in 172 popular online porn films, found forty-three per cent of the films they analysed contained physical violence such as forced gagging or forced vaginal penetration, or degradation such as ejaculation on a woman's face. Latina and Asian women were the most frequent recipients of violent behaviour.

Unlike the stranger elements of sexual fantasy, some believe that there is a link between watching violent porn and some viewers being accepting of violence against women. A 2011 study of nearly 3,000 American men, which asked them more than 300 questions about porn consumption and attitudes towards violence against women, concluded that, for men with a propensity towards antisocial behaviour, acts of aggression in porn 'when primed repeatedly, may result in the chronic accessibility of attitudes that minimise the responsibility of men who commit acts of aggression against women and may generally reinforce the acceptance of dominating, controlling and perhaps even violent acts of aggression against women'.

Naomi Wolf writes about this in *Vagina: A New Autobiography*, pointing out that many men try to stop watching porn, as using extreme, violent and degrading sex on screen as a way to get off does not exactly make them feel good about themselves. She thinks women are not immune to this either.

> *Female sexual response is adapting to male-porn's pacing – with consequent problems for women in libido and arousal under less intense sexual triggers, and to the detriment of both genders' sexuality and sense of connection.*

This is sad because a sense of connection is who we are, and at the very least, is often the starting point of great sex.

Hang on a minute, Hotbed. You are beginning to sound like Mary Whitehouse* now ...

Just to be clear, we're not suggesting a total ban on all porn. We don't even want a ban on hardcore porn.

To us it's like banning all processed food because of obesity, or outlawing alcohol because some people are alcoholics. Should we ban all hook-ups and relationships because there are sex and love 'addicts'? A little flutter on the horses isn't a reason to ban all gambling. Most people who watch porn can take it or leave it. They watch it just to enjoy it, and it has no bearing on how they treat other people or how they feel about themselves. It helps them masturbate, end of story.

So what we really don't like is the idea that young people watching porn are using it as the main source of their sex education. We want them to know that there is more to shagging than meets the eye.

---

*The British woman who in the Seventies and Eighties campaigned against sex, swearing and violence on television, and what she saw as the slackening of Christian morals of the UK as a result.

WHY IT'S A BIT SHIT THAT MAINSTREAM HETEROSEXUAL PORN RARELY DEPICTS GENUINE FEMALE PLEASURE

It's a myth that women want more romance in their porn and a soft lens — a Mills & Boon narrative with someone in black tie playing piano in the background — but wouldn't it be nice for the clitoris to play a part in some of the women's orgasms in porn? Eighty per cent of the orgasms, say, as in real life? Threeways, vigorous anal sex, being spunked on by your 'stepbrother' ... we're guessing they don't make the average woman particularly aroused.

In porn, there just isn't the same level of variety offered up to women: narratives that are clitoris-centric, that worship this amazing piece of the female anatomy, that give it the same status as the penis and its damn mission to *penetrate every woman in every way imaginable*.

Could it be that delicious, genuine orgasms are not 'showy' enough to be shown on screen in a sexy way and so the theatrics of porn sex have taken over? Are young men raised on mainstream porn expecting women to groan at the sight of their penis, and who then feel disappointed when they don't, and yet don't realise that you have to touch the clitoris for this to happen. And not only touch it but caress it, treat it tenderly.

Love it as your best friend.

Is it at least worth a conversation?

HAVING A CONVERSATION ABOUT PORN

When people (lawmakers, pundits, your elderly relatives, us at the beginning of this chapter) talk about porn — and admonish it for wrecking young minds, relationships and society — they are talking about hardcore, mainstream porn. This paints the entire industry with the same brush, with the conclusion that it is either a *good* thing or a *bad* thing (normally the latter).

This makes debate difficult, because banishing all porn means banishing all kinds of sexy images: from saucy postcards to erotic novels to feminist porn to sex toy tutorials on YouTube. It would be quite hard to draw the line.

And, if we're being very fair and honest, can we really argue that there is a huge difference between the female fantasies we talked about earlier, and the fantasies which often play out in mainstream porn? The common themes in both are taboo/forbidden encounters: think therapist and stepmum; control and domination; voyeurism; servicing people who are desperate for some lovin'; being lusted after, adored and pleasured by someone who requires not much input from you, and so on.

Is it fair to defend female fantasies yet cry, 'Hang on a minute, have we let this porn thing go a bit too far?'. In the same way that all food in moderation can be a good thing (who wants never to have a slice of birthday cake again, or to get an oven pizza after a long and stressful day?), can watching five minutes of standard porn every so often when you want a quick way to get the horn be a good thing too?

Yes ... but in the same way that we need to keep an eye on the food industry and how it markets and produces food, so we should keep an eye on the porn industry.

As humans, we are programmed to go for the easiest, quickest and most satisfying option. This is why when we're peckish, we are more likely to go for the Hobnob rather than bother to peel an orange. It's why we scroll through Instagram rather than read a long article or a book, and it's why we like to comment or focus on what someone looks like rather than engage with what they are saying.

People who make money know this, and often manipulate the depressing predictability of human nature to make more money. In tech, developers build in easy rewards such as 'likes' and 'shares' to give us little happy lifts every time we pick up our phones, thus keeping us hooked.

Fast food companies know that making cheap, easy-to-eat food with salty or sugary hits will mean that we can't resist. Porn bigwigs know that by making porn easy to access and immediately gratifying, we will return to their sites time and time again. This is documented nicely in Jon Ronson's podcast series *The Butterfly Effect,* which explores the building of Pornhub and all its repercussions.

So, even though it is seriously uncool to criticise porn, we think it's healthy to question everything, including the porn industry, how it works and how we, as customers, interact with it.

What we *can* do is change the narrative around porn, educate people about porn, and big up the alternatives to mainstream porn.

This is a call to arms (and hands, and fingers ...) and we need your help.

The Hot Hotbed Porn Manifesto

YOUNG PEOPLE SHOULD BE EDUCATED
ABOUT PORN

We believe that this should happen at home and at school.

We deal with sex education earlier in this book, but it's crucial that young people are told about the porn industry, about how it is filmed and how there are different kinds of porn, and how problematic some mainstream, male-gaze porn can be. They should be told how to get help if they see something that confuses them, or frightens them, or if they are being pressured to watch porn or film themselves in a pornographic way.

Parents should not be afraid not only to be open about porn (how about an 'in our day we couldn't watch porn on demand and had to settle for watching the sexy parts of *Eurotrash* and try to block out the comedy voiceovers'? That'll go down well).

It should also be made clear to young people that sex in real life is different, that it can and should be loving, tender, pleasurable for both parties, and doesn't normally involve a giant schlong and an entire cheerleading team (or penetrating everything, all the time, all day long).

ADULTS SHOULD BE EDUCATED ABOUT PORN

We're guessing that most of you reading this book did not grow up at a time when porn was as easily accessible as it is today, i.e. for free and on your mobile phone. It's not just young people who need to know more about the porn industry and its alternatives, we all have learning to do too.

Jon Ronson's *The Butterfly Effect* is a good place to start as well as *Pornland*. (Some more books and long reads are recommended in our Resources section.)

WE SHOULD TALK ABOUT IT

There's no point pretending that porn is going away. We are visual creatures who respond to tits, cocks and dirty talk. And while there are plenty of scenarios in which talking about your experience of porn is not appropriate (NCT classes, job interviews, your company's AGM), we do believe that talking about something banishes shame and spreads information: the more we talk about something, the more we learn.

THE PORN INDUSTRY SHOULD BE REGULATED

Like any industry. And, in fact, what bothers us about porn is largely what bothers us about many industries. We would enjoy porn a lot more if we knew that there was diversity at the top (we also know that, as with any industry, the output would be better if this was the case). We would like it if the stars were paid a bigger share of the profits that they help to generate.

The International Union of Sex Workers campaigns for fair rights for their members: for their right to work safely; be protected by the laws of their country; and to work in the industry without stigma. Hear hear. We really don't like that people can watch porn in public places. And we don't like that young people can find porn online when they are not even looking for it (a survey by the NSPCC found that more young people who had found porn online had found it accidentally than had sought it out themselves), and so we need to keep up the conversation, and not just be 'for' or 'against' porn.

THERE SHOULD BE GREATER VARIETY IN PORN

We can't pretend we're big fans of the rapey/humiliation/incesty-type porn. We also know that — as with fantasy — there is a difference between what turns us on to watch and what we actually want to do in real life.

We want to see more of the clitoris. We want to see it being treated right in porn, given a bit more of the limelight. We're a bit tired and jaded and aren't asking for much, hey?

So, let's enjoy porn, and know that alternative narratives are also available. These don't have to be soft-lens, romance scenarios where women swoon because a caped Prince Charming tells them they've got lovely eyes.

Feminist porn is great, but to make it a fair and thriving industry we need to support it: by promoting it, and paying for it.

Shall we put our money where our mouth (vulva?) is?

FEMINIST PORN

We like feminist porn because it acknowledges the fact that women are also turned on by sexual images and it tends to be made with female pleasure in mind too.

A bit like wearing a man's suit, the mainstream porn industry may sometimes work for us — for a bit of a laugh or a thrill — but could it be that it ultimately doesn't quite fit? Short of alternatives, women are flocking to gay male-on-male porn as an alternative. Pornhub reported that thirty-seven per cent of gay male porn is viewed by women. 'Pussy licking', 'lesbian scissoring' and 'lesbian threesomes' are also popular search terms for women (although so is 'gang bang') which suggests that we want to see a greater variety of sexual acts and practices which might feel good to us, as well as the odd dip into gang-banging.

For ladies who enjoy a good visual, we recommend looking up feminist porn films which offer another good alternative to the mainstream.

Feminist porn is characterised by all, or some, of the following:

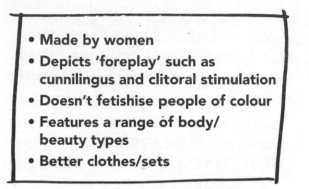

- **Made by women**
- **Depicts 'foreplay' such as cunnilingus and clitoral stimulation**
- **Doesn't fetishise people of colour**
- **Features a range of body/ beauty types**
- **Better clothes/sets**

If you like the sound of this, look up the work of film-makers such as Petra Joy, Erika Lust or Jennifer Lyon Bell. Erotic boutique Coco de Mer also makes sexy films that we think are *hot*. Last but not least, there is a site called Make Love Not Porn where you can pay to watch films that real couples have made for the site. They don't class themselves as a porn site, for this reason, but the films are pretty sexy all the same.

It must be said that certain radical feminists (Gail Dines included) don't like even feminist porn, as they say that any commodification of the female body is a patri-archal act. If you are interested in this debate, there is a brilliant transcript of a conversation between pornographer and artist Annie Sprinkle and anti-porn radical feminist Mae Tyme on Sprinkle's website. The link is in our Resources list.

'GUY: SO ... WHAT DO YOU DO FOR FUN? ME: I REALLY ENJOY FLIRTING ALL NIGHT THEN COMING HOME ALONE, TO MY COUCH, WHERE I MASTURBATE IN SOLITUDE, TURNED ON BY AN ALTERNATE LIFE IN WHICH I'M BRAVER AND MORE ENTITLED TO MEN'S BODIES. YOU? *SIPS DIET COKE*'

Michaela Coel

AN XXX HOTBED PORN FILM

We see a woman enter a bedroom. She has a beautiful body but it's also a body that we can identify with (for us, it's Lena Dunham in *Girls*, but magically, the film you are watching stars someone whose body you relate to). There's a mysterious man sitting on the bed (he's not on his iPad and is giving the woman his undivided attention).

The bedroom is tastefully decorated with old vintage furniture, retro wallpaper and a four-poster bed that is possibly Habitat (when it was still pricey and before it became part of Homebase). There's definitely a Diptique candle on the go (the one that smells like musky old churches but is strangely sexy).

The woman is wearing lingerie that looks like it might be Agent Provocateur and is definitely NOT a red thong. The soundtrack playing in the background is by The Kills (or another moody, sexy band).

'I want to make you come,' the man says seductively, looking the woman up and down (in a way that is deeply sexy and not like he's sizing up a prize heifer).

He undresses the woman slowly. He is stripped down to his underwear now too. He kisses her while she smokes a cigarette (because in this alternative porn reality, smoking does not give you cancer) and makes very little effort - possibly because she's had a long boring day at work and can't be bothered to do much.

He goes down on her for a good fifteen minutes (adjust time accordingly to suit your tastes). At the same time, he massages her nipples and whispers about how amazing she is, how beautiful her body is, how he has just bought her

a gift voucher for Harvey Nichols
because he knows there's a jumper on
the website that she likes, and she
deserves it because she's the most
precious person in the world.

She orgasms because he has NOT IGNORED
HER CLITORIS COMPLETELY.

He is wild with lust at having brought
about this amazing orgasm. They are
both steaming with excitement. She
gives him an appreciative blow job
which he most certainly did not ask for
by thrusting her head in the direction
of his crotch. They have a hot fuck
which is only low-to-middling athletic
and lasts as long as it takes for
the sweet potato wedges on downstairs
to cook.

He asks if she fancies anything else
and she says, 'That was amazing but, no
thanks. I might have a small nap
before dinner.'

She admires his bum and his back as
he walks past - now wearing the same
tasteful underpants that are definitely
not BRIGHT YELLOW/the type worn by a
Venice Beach muscle man in 1987.

She lights another cigarette and
manages to look smouldering, thoughtful
and empowered at the same time.

The End.

DURING PARTNERED SEX, WHICH PHYSICAL ACTIVITIES ARE MORE LIKELY TO BRING YOU TO THE POINT OF ORGASM?

1,209 responses

61.5%

Oral sex

58.5%

Fingering

50.7%

Masturbation

47.6%

Vibrating sex toy

45%

Vaginal penetration

29.7%

Nipple stimulation

11.3%

Anal play e.g.. fingering or licking

5.5%

Dildo style sex toy

We asked the same of orgasms during masturbation and the top answers were 'finger(s) on clitoris', 'vibrating sex toy' and 'nipple stimulation' in that order.

Coming Together
and Other Lies

11

LISA

I first had intercourse on the night Pretty Woman *was showing on TV. I can't say there were any similarities between what happened in my then-boyfriend's bedroom and what I saw on screen. I wasn't wearing a cut-out dress and thigh-high boots, I wasn't being paid to have sex, I didn't have a gold condom, even though I would have liked one, I wasn't treated to strawberries and champagne the morning after, but there definitely was kissing on the lips, unlike in the film.*

There was less sex on TV in the Nineties than there is today, so it was slim pickings when it came to my screen sex education. Nonetheless, watching Pretty Woman, Four Weddings and a Funeral, 9½ Weeks, Cocktail *and other big hits of that era, I did conclude that sex should include one or more of the following: a simultaneous, screaming orgasm; a buxom naked woman bouncing around the room/hotel suite/waterfall; a man who manages to hide his penis under a sheet or in his pants the entire time.*

I've now been having sex for two decades and I can't say that any of the above have come true.

Instead, there has been: other people walking in by accident; awkward conversations about what protection to use and when we last got tested; the constant worry of being overheard by neighbours/flatmates; faked orgasms; wet patches; and foreplay which lasts longer than an entire feature film.

Maybe these things would have been tricky to fit into the plot of Pretty Woman, *but still …*

TV is a mainstay of entertainment. We'd like to pretend that we're go-getters with diaries packed full of activism, activity and anal play, but the reality is that we spend the majority of our lives either in the playground, at our laptops staring into the middle distance or slumped on the sofa watching TV. Just like most other people.

Sex has become more prevalent on our TV screens. It's gone from something that was only seen very late at night in arty Channel 4 films, to something that's featured in every drama series we watch. And more sex is a good thing, right? We're no longer a nation of prudes who write letters of complaint because we've seen a bum or a pair of boobs. This surely is something to celebrate.

However, does watching all this sex make us more likely to feel aroused, engaged, empowered, sexy and to fancy a shag, or does the sex we see in the cinema and on TV feel unrealistic, demotivating, rose-tinted and clichéd? This is a key question, and we'd argue that more often than not, the answer is the latter.

A constant exposure to the same images (woman in ecstasy, woman's boobs, male bum pumping up and down, woman in ecstasy, more boob, couple coming together) not only shapes our perceptions of what 'good sex' looks like, it can also make us feel mighty boring. Dare we say it ... jaded ... maybe even nostalgic for a bit of *Dynasty*-style action when Alexis and Dex Dexter would clamber into a bubbling jacuzzi, and we'd cut straight to a shot of fireworks accompanied by a sexy saxophone solo?

What we love about the Netflix era of television is that we can watch what we want when we sit down (*Orange Is the New Black*, *Girls*, *GLOW*), rather than having to put up with whatever happens to be showing (usually *MasterChef*, *Blue Bloods or The One Show*).

As we get older, we're getting pickier, and for this reason we are thrilled at the emergence of a wave of brilliant, diverse writing for TV drama. When everyone sits at the table — when networks start bringing in more women, people of colour and members of the LGBTQIA community into the writers' room — the output becomes more nuanced, more interesting and more worthy of our time.

But we still have a long way to go. A 2018 survey by the University of California which looked at 200 films and 2,100 television shows released in 2015–2016 found that, despite some advances, women and people of colour were still underrepresented on both sides of the camera (despite proof that films with diverse casts do well at the box office).

You don't need us to go on about this: just a quick flick through the film and TV listings will tell you all you need to know on the topic.

HOW WHITE MEN ARE STILL SHAPING OUR VISUAL IMAGERY, EVEN IF WE *DO* HAVE A COUPLE OF GREAT FEMALE CREATIVE FORCES OUT THERE

We're not knocking white men, but the problem with an industry which gives white men all the storytelling power is that all the stories belong to, well, white men.

It shouldn't be groundbreaking to say the word 'clitoris' and explain what it does on terrestrial television in America but, when it was said during an episode of *Crazy Ex-Girlfriend*, it did indeed make headlines.

It shouldn't be noteworthy that a film features a love scene between a middle-aged black woman and a middle-aged white man but, when the 2018 film *Widows* opened with Viola Davis and Liam Neeson kissing in bed, Davis told the *Guardian*:

> *For me, that is something you'll not see this year, last year, the year before that. That is, a dark-skinned woman of colour, at fifty-three years old, kissing Liam Neeson. Not just kissing a white man: Liam Neeson, a hunk. And kissing him romantically, sexually.'*

Unless you are a peeping Tom or into dogging, you don't get to see other people having sex very often, and so what you see on screen really matters (we haven't written a chapter on dogging in this book, but let us know if it's something you'd like to know more about and we'll tackle it in our next one perhaps).

The thing is, it really matters that so much screen sex is told from the point of view of a man. We've touched on the term 'the male gaze' earlier in the book, but it's worth exploring here in depth. It was coined by Laura Mulvey in 1975 in her essay 'Visual Pleasure and

Narrative Cinema', which, if it could be distilled into two key sentences, would be the following:

> *Traditionally, the woman displayed [...] functions [...] as erotic object for the spectator within the auditorium [...] A woman performs within the narrative, the gaze of the spectator and that of the male characters in the film are neatly combined.*

The male gaze is essentially a masculine, heterosexual perspective – a way of representing women as sexual objects for the pleasure of the characters within the film and the male viewer sitting at home. You can see examples of it in photography, film – just about every cultural artefact you come across and once you become aware of it, it is almost impossible to become unaware. It's just the way we see the world as a whole, and it makes it difficult for women to define their own gaze and sexual appetite without focusing on what she and other women look like sexually. Representation matters.

'IT'S A STRUGGLE EVERY DAY TO GET PEOPLE TO INVEST FINANCIALLY IN PORTRAYALS OF WOMEN THAT AREN'T SATISFYING TO STRAIGHT WHITE MEN.'

Jill Soloway

Furthermore, men creating narratives might for instance have a limited understanding of female pleasure, and thus you often see the clichéd hetero-sexual white couple thrashing around in bed, having traditional penetrative intercourse until they both come to a noisy and coordinated orgasm.

As we already know, only twenty per cent of women can climax in this way, so isn't it strange that this 'vision' of sex still persists? And any women in that eighty per cent camp will know that watching this kind of sex and orgasm on screen contributes to that crushing sense of failure and questioning of what is normal. Simi-larly, couples coming together happens on screen far more than it does in real life. A survey of 4,400 people by sex toy company Lovehoney found that the average couple orgasms together once every three times they have sex. And in a Czech study, ten per cent of women and eight per cent of men in a sample of more than 1,500 people said they had never experienced a simultaneous orgasm with a sexual partner, compared to sixteen per cent of women and men who said they 'always or almost always do'.

We see athletic positions that rarely reflect the reality of everyday sex: Anniki was disappointed to discover that *9½ Weeks* starring Mickey Rourke and Kim Basinger did *not* reflect the sex lives of your average couple (have you ever been blindfolded and fed an array of sensual foods from the fridge?).

We don't need all screen sex to show empowered, sexual women having the greatest sex of their lives (as in feminist porn). What we want to see is *real* sex and, if it can't be real, we want it to be interesting: funny, imaginative, varied. Sex can be hot, heartbreaking, crushing, boring, athletic, lazy, and so many other adjectives. We want to see sex which mirrors what's actually happening in bedrooms and backseats across the world. We want to see sex which doesn't perpetuate tired and sometimes damaging myths about sex and sexuality.

HOW TO ANALYSE THE SEX YOU SEE ON SCREEN FOR THE GREATER GOOD

Have you heard of the Bechdel Test? It is named after the graphic novelist Alison Bechdel, who devised the test which first appeared in her comic strip *Dykes to Watch Out For*. It's a neat way of becoming more aware of how female characters are portrayed on screen. To pass the Bechdel Test, a film has to show two named female characters talk to each other about a topic which *isn't* men. It's amazing how many films fail this test and, like the male gaze, once you start to be aware of it, it's hard not to be on the alert while watching movies.

There is a similar test proposed by the writer Nikesh Shukla which examines whether there are two named people of colour who talk to each other for five minutes about an issue which isn't race. These tests have their limitations, and just passing the test does not make a great work of art, and there are many great works which fail. Similarly, some films just can't pass these tests because of a historical or geographical setting (although we have to question why so many works like this are made and what that tells us about history and who commissions and funds films). A good example of the limits of this test is the song 'Baby Got Back' by Sir Mix-a-Lot: while not a film, this passes because two women talk about another woman's great butt. Then the original *Star Wars* films fail because, despite how wonderful Princess Leia is, the poor love doesn't get to talk to any other women.

Nevertheless, tests like this are a useful way of using data to challenge what we see on screen, and so we propose the Hotbed Test: a checklist of things we like to see when sex is seen on screen. To pass the test, and because we acknowledge that we still have a long way to go, we propose that a work just needs to meet two of these criteria in order to pass, although the funny thing is that, when a film or TV show passes point one, it tends to pass several of the other points too. This is the future ...

SEX ON SCREEN: THE HOTBED TEST

1. Has the film/TV show been written/directed/ produced by a woman, person of colour or some-one from the LGBTQIA community?

2. Is contraception mentioned or shown? Wouldn't it be nice to see couples broach the question about being tested for STIs and/or asking where the condoms are?

3. Does the clitoris get a look in? The clitoris is the most underplayed character in Hollywood. We would like to see more oral sex, more foreplay, and more mentions of the clitoris, please.

4. If it's bad sex, is it acknowledged as bad sex? We don't want every sex scene to be perfect. There can be bad sex, of course, because bad sex happens all the time and is part of our experience, but is it depicted as bad sex? Is there an eye roll or a conversation with a friend about it afterwards, or something clever with editing or camera angles or soundtrack that makes it apparent it is so?

5. Is there nudity equality? We love naked women, but we also love naked men. If there are boobs and bushes on display, some sexy backs, erections and some (straight) girl gaze would be great, thank you.

6. Is consent clear? We don't need to see a contract being filled out, but we would like to see some screen depictions of how you establish clear consent. And when it isn't clear, is it framed as a bad thing or not mentioned?

7. If body-shaming exists, it is questioned? As we have discussed, low body confidence can play a key role in our ability to enjoy sex, and the male gaze and its resultant body fascism is partly to blame for this. There is a lot of body-shaming on screen, unfortunately, and it's often seen as funny. Why are the old/

ugly/thin/fat characters often the figure of fun or the 'loser' of the story? Let's move on from these lazy stereotypes.

8. Is there racial stereotyping and fetishisation? True progress is when all characters are as three-dimensional and developed as the white men.

9. Does the woman have sexual agency? Is she active or passive in bed? Does she initiate sex and/or stop it? Does she talk about sex without blushing? Does she masturbate for her own pleasure?

10. Are there other forms of realism in the scene? These are the unexpected, funny, strange and emotional things that can happen during sex which we don't see enough of: think of a couple starting to have sex and then stopping halfway because they're too tired, or when sex happens with socks on, or if there's erectile dysfunction or lubrication is needed or someone steps on Lego on their way to the bed. More real sex, please.

Here are some movies and shows with sex scenes that pass the test by breaking the mould and reflecting, even just a little bit, some of our reality:

TRANSPARENT This series about a Jewish family with three grown-up children and a father who transitions to a woman (informed by writer Jill Soloway's experience of having a transitioning parent), shows heterosexual and LGBT sex in many forms, in a way which always feels natural and not shoehorned. We like it because diverse characters we care about have all kinds of diverse sex: from missionary to threesomes and yet, bizarrely, this sex isn't always central to the plot.

DON'T LOOK NOW An oldie but a goodie. The sex scene between Donald Sutherland and Julie Christie's characters — the first time their characters have sex after losing a child — is so realistic (a bit awkward, messy but very intimate) that people thought they'd had sex for real. It was one of the first times cunnilingus was shown in mainstream cinema.

GIRLS So much to love in Lena Dunham's landmark drama, namely showing bodies of different sizes (albeit mainly all white, cis- and able), more 'specialist' acts such as rimming, and shower sex between an older couple going wrong.

GREY'S ANATOMY Shonda Rhimes did 'colourblind' casting for this series, which meant she didn't have a racial profile in mind for the initial characters, and a diverse, interesting cast was appointed as a result. This series has sexy people doing important things, and has made people less afraid of talking about their 'vajajays', a term which was coined on this show. Amen.

I LOVE DICK Another Jill Soloway venture, this adaptation of the book of the same name is excellent at showing different manifestations of female desire, from the standing-in-a-tiny-trailer-kitchen lesbian hook-up, to the breathless lust Katherine Heigl's character has for the titular Dick, which forms the main thrust of the story. Bonus points for showing period sex.

GLOW Not only is there a solid, loving relationship between two black characters (2019 and this is noteworthy), but the raw sexuality and diversity of bodies on this show, about Eighties cable show *The Gorgeous Ladies of Wrestling*, is empowering, and clearly what happens when you have a diverse production team and majority female cast.

FLEABAG Phoebe Waller-Bridge's play-turned-TV series wins a Hotbed award for showing the title character masturbate to Barack Obama videos on YouTube.

THE SHAPE OF WATER Not only does Sally Hawkins' character initiate hot, underwater sex in this fantasy film by Guillermo del Toro and Vanessa Taylor, but we also see her have a nice wank as part of her daily routine.

Snogging:
We Need It,
We Want It

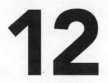

ANNIKI

The word 'snogging' is said to have originated in British India in the Forties. When I looked it up online, the definition I found is 'kissing and cuddling amorously'.

However, in my book snogging means the following:

A kiss with tongues.

A kiss with tongues that feels rude and indecent.

A kiss with tongues that feels rude and indecent and goes on for a long time.

It also (sadly) feels like something that's gone out of fashion. Even among spring chickens.

Statistics from a survey of 27,000 people conducted by the Florida Atlantic University suggest that millennials are less likely to be having sex than young adults thirty years ago. The younger generation is less promiscuous (also taking less drugs, drinking less), but does this also mean that they're snogging less too?

If snogging were a sport, I'd be an Olympic champion. My core snogging years were the late Eighties/early Nineties. My school friend Kate drew a cartoon line-up of all the boys I snogged in one year (twenty-five in total). I still have this drawing in the loft. I was looking for the old Moses basket some months back, and found it in a box next to a Morcheeba album. This fading piece of scrap paper made me sad for two reasons:

I don't snog anymore

I miss it.

Snogging in my teens was an activity much like going ice-skating or watching a film but more fun than both of those put together.

The benefits were pretty clear too ...

- *Snogging didn't mean SEX: it was an activity in its own right.*
- *It was pure, unadulterated, glorious foreplay: an opportunity to be sexy without the fear of pregnancy/sore vagina from vigorous fingering etc.*
- *It didn't mean commitment. One evening my three friends and I snogged the same boy. There was a spirit of camaraderie between us and no jealousy.*
- *It was a laugh (this chapter is not about bad snogs but let's be clear, there were those too, of course, and they were rarely fun).*

I've snogged in the back of nightclubs. On the top deck of buses. In Pizza Hut booths (the salad bar was the height of luxury back then). In the cinema watching He Man – Masters of The Universe. *Behind Camden market.*

I've snogged boys who had quiffs. Boys who looked a tiny bit like Michael Hutchence. Boys who had braces on their teeth. Boys who sprayed Lynx deodorant down their 501s. Boys with tattoos. Boys who smelt like fried onions. Boys who danced like MC Hammer. The list goes on ...

Like a lover of fine wine, a bon viveur, a truffle-hunting piglet, I came to understand there were different types of snoggers. The round-and-round-like-a-washing-machine snogger. The serial dribblers. The fixated-on-giving-you-a-love-bite snogger. And the I'm-shoving-my-hand-into-your-pants-without-any-warning sort (to be avoided). Pure snog-meisters were prized the most.

There's a big part of me that hopes that despite the growth of social media, the relentless documentation of every part of our lives, teens feeling under pressure to present themselves in a positive light, pushing back against previous generations who've behaved badly and refuse to grow old, the need to be perfect, popular, not be judged ... well, I hope those teens are still snogging.

I'm keenly aware that I sound a bit like the misty-eyed grandma in a Werther's Original advert, rocking on my chair, chomping on my dentures, a blanket on my knees, ruing the way things have changed. But I do feel nostalgic about snogging because it tends to be one of those enjoyable things that goes on the back burner as we age and grow up.

It's time to bring more snogging back into our lives.

We all have those positive (and, let's face it, not so positive) memories of snogging. It's foreplay in its purest form (and while we're at it, dare we say that we rather miss some of those steamy 'dry humping' sessions too?). Snogging doesn't need to lead to penetration: it can just be an all-engrossing activity in itself.

We snogged a lot in our teens. We snogged our partners when we first met. We then continued to snog them as the relationship grew and matured. But ... eventually...

The snogging dried up.

This isn't true for everyone, but many of our listeners and readers tell us that their snogging days seem to be over.

Yes, times have changed. Yes, the older among us may want to sit down and have a soft drink when we're out on the town. Yes, perhaps we think that some of the clothes in Topshop are silly and won't keep us warm in winter. But that doesn't mean we have to hang up our snogging shoes for ever.

'I AM A STRONG BELIEVER IN KISSING BEING VERY INTIMATE, AND THE MINUTE YOU KISS, THE FLOODGATES OPEN FOR EVERYTHING ELSE.'

Jennifer Lopez

Snogging tends to get lost in the day-to-day interaction of long-term relationships, perhaps because, as time goes on, the novelty of physical intimacy wears off, or maybe because we know that sex is a probability when we're in a happy relationship, rather than the thrilling 'will-we-won't-we?' ceremony of the dating days. There are loads of other gestures and touches that get kicked to the kerb too: hair stroking, massage, caressing, playful pinching, flirtatious conversations, playing footsie, innuendo ... These are often the things that make sex playful and fun, in other words, not all about the actual shagging.

There is no law that says only teenagers are allowed to snog (if they are still snogging at the rate that we did, that is). What's more, it offers a raft of benefits. It brings you closer to your partner. It releases oxytocin, dopamine and serotonin into the body (which boost your mood). It can even tone up your facial muscles (so forget Botox and all that shit).

Don't relegate snogging to a dusty cartoon drawing that lives in the attic. Bring it on!

HOW TO GET SNOGGING BACK INTO YOUR LIFE

'But how do I get snogging back into my repertoire?' we hear you cry. 'I miss it. I want it. I love it. I want to snog my son's music teacher. I want to snog that train driver. I want to snog **EVERYONE**.' (Oh, are you ovulating by the way?)

Fair question. Here are our Hotbed Tips to help build more snogs into your relationship.

1. For a start, snogging requires a certain amount of letting down your guard. It feels peculiarly intimate: more intimate than having full-blown sex. Isn't that weird? Kick things off with a 'warm-up to snogging' week. Kiss your partner more often. When they leave the house, try kissing them on the lips rather than shouting at them that they've shoved a load of polystyrene packaging in with the recycling.

2. Try introducing a few more physically intimate gestures. Maybe pinch their bum or stroke their arm. Remember the little things you did to one another when you first met. Talk about these things (you can always have this conversation while driving so it doesn't feel too intimate and it's better than arguing over the faulty satnav). This is about creating a greater sense of physical intimacy between the two of you.

3. Then, when the moment feels right ... snog.

    Maybe you've had a couple of glasses of wine.

    Maybe you're at the bus stop. Don't overthink it. Just give it a go.

And if you're sixteen and reading this, get out and snog and snog and snog. As Róisín Murphy of Moloko sang in the Noughties dance classic, 'Give up yourself unto the moment. The time is now.' Also a good song to kiss to, incidentally.

In our youth there were certain songs that helped set the mood when it came to heavy kissing and all that jazz. We've put together a short playlist of our favourite tracks. Play these at home to help bring back those vibes, and get ready to pucker up:

THE HOTBED
SNOGGING PLAYLIST

'IF I WAS YOUR GIRLFRIEND' by Prince
(in fact, pretty much anything by Prince)

'COME TO DADDY' by Aphex Twin
this might be more of an angry session with an
ex–boyfriend

'MAPS' by the Yeah Yeah Yeahs
crying and snogging = bliss

'WAITING FOR THE NIGHT' by Depeche Mode
Dave Gahan in leather trousers: what more
do you need?

'LET'S GET IT ON' by Marvin Gaye
our parents snogged to this, but that doesn't
make it wrong

'FRENCH KISS' by Little Louis
go for the 12–inch version

'CLOSE TO ME' by The Cure
a classic

'MAKE IT WIT CHU' by Queens of the Stone Age
no explanation needed

'CREEP' by TLC
brings back those authentic 'Saturday night at
Streatham Ice Rink' vibes

'BEAUTIFUL GIRL' by Inxs
the lyrics alone make this is a snogging anthem

'TOUCH ME, TEASE ME' by Case ft. Foxy Brown
this song is so damn sexy it'll make you deranged
with lust

I Blame the
Hormones

13

LISA

I'm wearing compression stockings and a pantyliner the size of a mattress. My knickers come up to my waist and there's a chance I haven't had a shower for forty-eight hours.

At my breast is a tiny baby who has finally latched on to feed after a good thirty minutes of struggling (him) and crying (both of us). My shoulders are so tense that stretching them out nearly winds me, and my sleep has been so broken that I'm beginning to lose the concept of time. My husband, caring, loving, wonderful, comes up the stairs and, as I'm feeding, kisses me on the cheek.

I am so repelled by this kiss that I want him to leave the room.

At that point, I wouldn't even mind if he kept on walking and never came back. I think about moving to a female-only commune where I can drink herbal tea and join a breastfeeding collective so some other women can help breastfeed my baby.

I don't think I'll ever have sex again, and neither do I want to.

While having a baby can give some women a wonderful, magnetic 'glow', for most of us it is a deeply unsexy time. And it's not just because of the ugly 'compression' stockings, the pantyliners and the greasy hair. In the postnatal period your hormones play havoc with your body and your brain, and make you behave in a way which you don't recognise.

Alas, it's not only after childbirth that we can wind up feeling like we'll never want to have sex ever again. Like the most ruthless of puppet-masters, or the most villainous of Shakespeare villains, our hormones can play havoc with our libido. Hormones pull the strings on our thoughts and our feelings from behind the scenes. They are potent, clever, manipulative little fuckers.

You see, though you may think you have free will and are the sole author of your own destiny, sometimes you are not. Remember that time you gave that brilliant speech which ended with rapturous applause and you thought it was all down to your genius and your comic timing, or that day on your post-exams girls' holiday to Magaluf when three different blokes asked to snog you and you thought it was all because of your Sun-In highlights and the alluring way you smoked a Benson & Hedges? Well, we have news for you: a lot of stuff that happens to you can partly be explained by — yes, you guessed it — hormones.

On the upside, hormones can also explain some of the stuff that might frustrate you about yourself. Like the days when you're tired and grumpy and you only mean to eat one jaffa cake, but you end up eating the whole packet. Or like when you spend all day telling your friends what a shitbag your ex-boyfriend is but then you end up having a drink, and booty-calling him anyway. Or when whomever you're shagging is great and doing all the right things but you just lie there stroking their back, not really enjoying yourself and not knowing why. **HORMONES**, girl. **HORMONES**.

Hey Hotbed, stop saying 'hormones' and start telling us about them, please!

For so long, 'hormones' was a word we used without really knowing what it meant. We would say, 'I'm feeling hormonal at the moment', while demolishing a packet of chocolate Hobnobs and we knew that being a teenager means having 'hormones flying around'. We had a vague concept that exercise boosts your endorphins, and that endorphins make you happy. But if you had turned around and asked us what a hormone was, we would have looked off to the middle distance, squinted our eyes and drawn a blank. Then we would have offered you a chocolate Hobnob and changed the subject.

But then we had babies and, when we were preparing for birth, in between wild sex dreams about Dave Grohl, we learnt about a hormone called oxytocin. Lisa recalls a particularly memorable antenatal class in which the teacher explained that oxytocin is needed to bring on labour contractions and to help push the baby out at birth, and that the conditions required to bring on oxytocin production were the same ones you might want while making love. Everyone got into groups to write a list of perfect love-making conditions such as a dark room and gentle or rhythmical music. One group clown wrote 'a bottle of wine', and so on.

Oxytocin is known as 'the love hormone', and it is released during sex, and during breastfeeding, and not only does it do practical things such as bring on contractions in birth, bring on vaginal lubrication during sex, or bring on milk production during breastfeeding, but it also helps promote bonding between humans.

When we set up the Hotbed Collective we were interested to find out more about hormones to understand why pregnancy and breastfeeding had had such an impact on our libido, and if there was anything we could do about it.

And if we were to have a conversation about what we learnt, it would go something like this:

A: [filing nails] So what are
hormones?

B: Hormones are naturally-
occurring chemicals which are
produced in the glands, and
transmitted via the blood to the
relevant organ, signalling the
body to make a change.

A: Stop there. What are glands?

B: We have a few, and they each
produce different hormones.

The pituitary gland, for example,
is in the brain, and it produces
hormones such as Follicle-stimulating hormone (FSH) which helps
trigger body changes in puberty.

The adrenal glands are in the kid-
neys, and they produce hormones
such as cortisol which helps us to
regulate stress.

The testicles are a gland and, in
male-bodied people, they produce
the hormone testosterone.

A: Oh I've heard of that one too.

B: It stimulates sperm production,
and hair growth on places such as
the chest and chin.

A: Doesn't it also make people
quite aggressive too?

B: It can do. Some studies have found that testosterone levels can rise during competitive sports games, and that people convicted of violent crimes have higher levels of the hormone.

A: And doesn't it make you want to have sex with that attractive dad in the playground when you've never actually thought of him in that way before?

B: That too. Female-bodied people produce testosterone too, in smaller amounts, and it can stimulate sexual desire in them too. Loss of sex drive in men can sometimes be explained by a dip in testosterone. And many trans women find that their sex drive changes as they undergo hormonal therapy, with a reduction in their testosterone signalling a move from the full-on horn to a gentler, but more fulfilling sexuality. Some trans men have found the opposite.

A: So how else can hormones affect my sex life?

B: In so many ways. For example, when you are breastfeeding, the milk-production hormone prolactin can cause a dip in sex drive, which makes sex after kids a bit tricky, especially when you don't understand what is happening to you. Babies, aside, when you have

```
sex with someone, the oxytocin
released in your body, which can
make you feel euphoric, can also
stay in your body for up to TWO
YEARS, which can sometimes explain
why you may feel attached to a
sexual partner long after you had
sex with them.

A: Hm, that sounds familiar.
*stops texting ex* Oh well, at
least I've had my kids now and
stopped breastfeeding. Hormones
can't interfere with my vagina
any longer, can they?

B: Well, actually, they can. As
women go through menopause, their
oestrogen and progesterone levels
change, which can lead to a loss
of sex drive and increased
vaginal dryness, which sounds like
terrible news but there are meas-
ures you can take to alleviate
these symptoms.

A: Ok, listen that's a bit of a
downer.  Also how come you're
suddenly the conversational equiv-
alent of a GCSE biology textbook?

B: Sorry. *eats Hobnob*
```

Blaming your hormones won't give you a free pass to behave in ways you wouldn't normally consider accept-able, but knowing how they affect your body and your moods can help you understand yourself, and allow you to go easy on yourself for feeling or acting in a certain way, or to get help when you might need it.

HOW TO GET THOSE HORMONES WORKING FOR YOU AND YOUR SEX LIFE

Here is a rundown of how your hormones can affect your sex, relationships and reproductive health at key stages of your life, from puberty to menopause. They do a lot more than this, but Hotbed's the name and sex is our game, so this is our angle. If you are interested in the topic, have a look in the Resources section for some good books on hormones more broadly, and how they affect you. You can also now find apps which track your cycles and hormonal levels in real time; armed with this information and how it might affect your body and mood, you can plan accordingly.

'THE PROBLEM WITH LOOKING IN THE MIRROR IS THAT YOU NEVER KNOW HOW YOU WILL FEEL ABOUT WHAT YOU SEE. SOMETIMES, WHEN MY HORMONES ARE OUT OF SYNC, I HAVE NO INTEREST IN THE MIRROR, AND IF I DO LOOK, I THINK EVERYTHING IS ALL WRONG. OTHER TIMES, I AM QUITE PLEASED WITH WHAT I SEE.'

Chimamanda Ngozi Adichie

PUBERTY

(or why you can't stop thinking about Ruby Rose/ Harry Styles/the new science teacher, and are also liable to explode with no warning)

WHAT HAPPENS: Follicle-stimulating hormone (FSH) and luteinising hormone (LH) travel via the blood to the ovaries to tell them to start producing oestrogen and progesterone, the so-called 'sex hormones' for women, which will trigger body changes to transform you, physically speaking, from a child to an adult.

WHAT'S NORMAL: Periods start; boobs grow; hips widen; voice drops; bad skin; mood swings; pubic hair growth; white vaginal discharge; weight gain; height gain. You may also start to experience sexual feelings, such as tingles or throbbing in your vulva.

HOW TO TREAT YOURSELF: With care! Puberty is a normal life change which we all go through. Remember to eat well and keep up your exercise and activity even, if you can bear it, during your period. Now is when you might want to start masturbating, and while this is an activity which happens in a private space such as your bedroom or bathroom, it is not shameful either, and experimenting with yourself is a natural and healthy thing. If you want to start experimenting sexually with someone else, this can be healthy too: as long as you are both over sixteen, and you consent to the activity. (See more on Consent p.108)

WHEN TO GET HELP: If you are feeling depressed or suffering from low self-esteem; if you have any discharge which smells bad or which isn't clear or white;

if your vulva feels itchy; if you are feeling overwhelmed with the emotional or physical changes. If you are feeling pressure to have physical contact with anyone you don't want to. If you have any questions or worries about pleasure, pregnancy, contraception or sexually transmitted diseases.

OVULATION

(or why 'No Diggity' by Blackstreet makes you twerk around the kitchen, and you get misty-eyed whenever a fit man walks past you in Lidl)

WHAT HAPPENS: Oestrogen and progesterone are at their peak, preparing the body for an egg to be fertilised. It is normally around day 9–15 of your menstrual cycle (with day 1 being the first day of your period), and is your most fertile period of the month.

WHAT'S NORMAL: Feeling horny; fuller boobs; glossier hair; confident, can-do attitude.

HOW TO TREAT YOURSELF: If you're trying for a baby, this is the best time to have sex. If you're not, this is still a good time to have sex, albeit with birth control, as you will have increased libido, a wetter vagina and will feel more sensitive to the touch and generally on fire. You can also maximise the can-do attitude by scheduling important events such as public speaking, a job interview, important meeting or date for these days.

WHEN TO GET HELP: If you bleed between periods; if you bleed after sex; if sex is painful.

BEFORE YOUR PERIOD

(or why you get really annoyed when someone jokes 'Oh, she must have her period')

WHAT HAPPENS: Oestrogen and progesterone levels drop suddenly, to signal to the body that the egg has not been fertilised, you are not pregnant, and that menstruation should start.

WHAT'S NORMAL: Achy boobs; mood swings; increased appetite; decreased sex drive and sensitivity.

HOW TO TREAT YOURSELF: Go easy on yourself. Eat regular, nutritious meals, have an early night, try to fit in some exercise. Some women find that the tension helps them to bring up things which are annoying them, others find that they are more short-tempered than normal and that they should avoid conflict at this time.

WHEN TO GET HELP: If your period is heavier or lighter than normal; if your periods become irregular or if they stop. If you find your mood swings hard to control.

THE CONTRACEPTIVE PILL

(or why do I not feel sexy yet I'm taking something to help me have sex?)

WHAT HAPPENS: Taking the combined pill, which contains artificial versions of oestrogen and progesterone, helps prevent pregnancy by stopping your ovaries from releasing an egg while also thickening the mucus of the cervix to make it more difficult for sperm to reach the egg, and thinning the womb lining so, if sperm was to reach an egg, it would be harder for it to implant and create a viable pregnancy.

WHAT'S NORMAL: Mood swings; nausea; a dip in sex drive; weight gain; headaches; sore boobs. Not exactly a sexy combination. But it also can make your periods lighter and less painful, and has some health benefits such as reducing the risk of cancer of the ovaries, womb and colon.

HOW TO TREAT YOURSELF: There is a bit of an irony in taking the pill because, although it is ninety-nine per cent effective in preventing pregnancy, its side effects can put you off sex completely. If you are having trouble getting in the mood for sex or masturbation, things such as sex toys, lube, sexy, mood-boosting activities such as massage, and affection for affection's sake can help rebuild desire. Remember, there are other contraception choices if the pill doesn't work for you.

WHEN TO GET HELP: If you are feeling depressed or anxious; if sex is painful or you can't orgasm any more; if your health situation changes such as you start smoking or getting migraines, or if your weight gain is excessive.

PREGNANCY

(or why am I up one minute and irritable the next? Shouldn't this be a fantastically happy time?)

WHAT HAPPENS: Oestrogen and progesterone stay high, to help your body grow the baby. Prolactin is produced to prepare you for breastfeeding. Relaxin helps relax your joints and muscles to make space for the growing baby. Oxytocin maintains your cervix for baby-holding, and prepares your body for birth.

WHAT'S NORMAL: Nausea and sickness; muscle ache; a 'blooming' feeling of wellbeing.

HOW TO TREAT YOURSELF: Pelvic floor exercises to help combat incontinence and painful sex. Sex and masturbation are safe during pregnancy, unless you have any complications, or if you are actually in labour, when infection is more likely. Regular, nutritious meals. Plenty of sleep.

WHEN TO GET HELP: If you are feeling depressed or not excited about the pregnancy; if you have any bleeding or spotting; if you find your moods to be uncontrollable; if you are wetting yourself or if sex is painful. *(Please note this is not an exhaustive list of red flags, but a few hormonal changes which may require further examination. If you have any worries at all related to your pregnancy, you should seek the advice of your health visitor, midwife or GP.)*

AFTER CHILDBIRTH

(or why do I cry into my dinner and get the sudden urge to throttle my partner?)

WHAT HAPPENS: Now you are no longer housing a baby inside you, oestrogen and progesterone are not needed in such high volumes, and they take a sudden dip after birth. Oxytocin can fluctuate, depending on factors such as how your labour was (a birth which goes to plan can cause a boost in the love hormone, a traumatic one can cause a dip), and whether or not you are breastfeeding. If you are breastfeeding, your body produces prolactin to help with milk production, and the elastin which allowed your body some flexibility to accommodate the baby is still in your system for several months.

WHAT'S NORMAL: Feeling loved up and as if all is well in the world at some moments, thanks to the oxytocin. But the dip in oestrogen and progesterone can cause the 'baby blues' roughly four days after birth, which may have you feeling low and teary. It's a confusing time! On a physical level, the prolactin from breast-feeding can make your sex drive nosedive, while the elastin will further weaken your pelvic floor muscles.

HOW TO TREAT YOURSELF: Like a Fabergé egg, in short. The postnatal period can be one of the most turbulent in a woman's life, due to the myriad physical and mental transitions you are going through. If there is ever a time to use your support networks: friends, family, neighbours, your local children's centre, your partner if you have one, and paid help if you can afford it, it is NOW. If anyone offers to help, enlist them to hold the baby while you catch up on sleep, ask them to make you a hot, nutritious meal or to batch-cook on your behalf. Keep up your fluids and eat well. Don't worry about your non-existent sex drive, you will get it back. Keep communicating with your partner if you have one, they will understand. Don't think that getting the all-clear for sex at your six-week check means that you have to get back in the sack again. Go at your pace, remember that you are a slave to rampant hormones, and think about maintaining affection and communication above sexy time. You will be a sex goddess again, but now is not your time. See the Cunnilingus and Snogging chapters for gentler alternatives to full-blown sex.

WHEN TO GET HELP: If you are feeling despairing and/or if you have lost your lust for life. If you feel as if you are losing a grip on reality or if you want to damage yourself or the baby in any way. The hormonal changes can trigger postnatal depression or postnatal psychosis, so it is very important that you see a GP or speak to a health visitor if this is the case.

THE PERIMENOPAUSE

(or why do I feel like I'm getting old and no one will ever want to have sex with me again?)

WHAT HAPPENS: As you approach menopause (usually in a woman's thirties or forties), oestrogen levels plummet to send a message to your reproductive system to start slowing down. Testosterone levels, which drop gradually after the production peak in your twenties, continue to decrease but do not stop completely. Once your body stops producing progesterone you are considered menopausal.

WHAT'S NORMAL: Hot flushes; mood swings; irritability; your periods slow down and stop (once you have missed twelve periods you are considered to have gone through the menopause); vaginal dryness; dip in sex drive; inflammation of the vagina (vaginal atrophy); weak pelvic floor.

HOW TO TREAT YOURSELF: It is now more important than ever to keep up those pelvic floor exercises (see our chapter on the pelvic floor for more information), be extremely kind to yourself, seek support and kinship among your friends around the topic, investigate lube and vaginal mousses to help restore moisture and help with sex and masturbation (Yes Organics is a good brand. See p.77). Masturbation can also help with boosting blood flow to the vulva area, lift mood and help keep you orgasmic.

WHEN TO GET HELP: If you are experiencing menopausal symptoms, it is a good idea to see your GP, who can confirm if it is the menopause using a blood test, and advise you on what medical treatments (such as HRT and/or hormone creams) and counselling/therapy is available, as well as being able to rule out other causes of the symptoms. (See Growing Old Disgracefully on p.293 for more information.)

Thanks, Hotbed, that's a lot of information to take in. Is me getting bored of reading and wandering off to check what's in the fridge also a symptom of my hormones?

Well, no, not really. And yes, it is a lot of information to take in, and yet we haven't even scratched the surface. What we wanted to do with this chapter is to cover some of the basics on our biology, because the more we understand about our bodies, and the interplay between our hormones and desire and sex, the closer we get to being orgasmic, empowered and altogether happier.

The Pelvic Floor:
Bear With Us

14

LISA

I'm pregnant with my second baby and being told from every direction to do my pelvic floor exercises. Then for various reasons I have a C-section scheduled and those pelvic floor exercises? Well, I don't need to do them, do I?

The baby is coming out via the sunroof, and so my vagina will remain as perky as before. Pelvic floor exercises are so boring, I only manage to remember to do them a) when someone mentions them to me or b) when I find myself with literally nothing else to do. Skip forward to when my son is here and I go to see my older son in his nursery Christmas concert.

I'm so proud I'm crying before I even sit down. We have been practising a lot and I've used an old pillow case and some red ribbon to make his 'Census Taker' outfit. I predict that in the course of the twenty-minute show, two children will cry, most of them will forget their words, one will try to escape, and three will wet themselves.

The opening song is adorable: cute baby faces smiling and singing, and waving to their mums. The narrator starts to speak, yelling 'Once upon a time in Bethlehem' so loudly into the microphone that we all startle, the naughty parents like me start laughing, and two children start crying.

On it goes, each child yelling one-note and seven notches too loudly into the microphone.

'Have you any room in this inn? How many people can you fit in?'

It's too much. I'm laughing so hard that the pew is convulsing and I am crying. Three children forget their words. One tries to escape. And I wet myself.

If, like Lisa, you think you are above doing your pelvic floor exercises, think again. *Unless* you are happy to be the kind of person who can't watch stand-up comedy without taking a waterproof seat protector, or hop onto the bouncy castle without issuing a flood warning. Look after your pelvic floor muscles and they will look after you. They can:

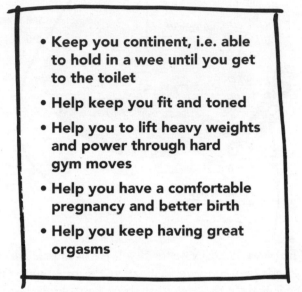

- **Keep you continent, i.e. able to hold in a wee until you get to the toilet**
- **Help keep you fit and toned**
- **Help you to lift heavy weights and power through hard gym moves**
- **Help you have a comfortable pregnancy and better birth**
- **Help you keep having great orgasms**

If none of the above is for you, skip to the next chapter. Otherwise, read on …

Like the clitoris, the pelvic floor is a part of our bodies which we hear about a lot, especially during pregnancy. Most of us, nevertheless, have no idea what it is, what it looks like or where it is. But the pelvic floor is important. So important, in fact, that if we could close the pay gap and fix the pelvic floor, women would have made very good inroads into equality with men. This is what the pelvic floor looks like:

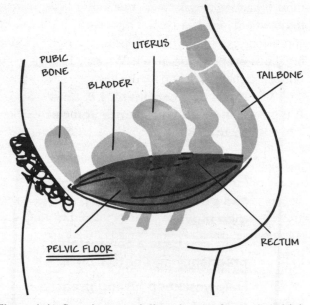

PUBIC BONE

UTERUS

BLADDER

TAILBONE

PELVIC FLOOR

RECTUM

The pelvic floor is essentially a layer of muscle which extends between your tailbone at the back and your pelvic bone at the front (just above your clitoris hood). In gym-instructor-speak, it is part of what is known as 'your core' and so when they bark stuff like, 'brace your core' or 'keep your core strong', they are referring to a box-like frame of muscle which has the diaphragm at the top (under your ribcage), the deep abs at the front, the back muscles at the back and the pelvic floor at the bottom.

Think of it as a protective hammock or sports bra, even, under your downstairs areas, which helps protect the bowels, bladder and uterus and keep them all in place. Unless you are a pilates devotee or an elite athlete, most of us don't really have much of an idea of what to do when a gym instructor barks at us to 'keep our core strong', or find it hard to locate the exact muscles he/she is even talking about. We usually do a vague buttock-clench and hope for the best.

It is great that the #fitfam care about the pelvic floor, but not so great when they don't take the time to explain *what it is exactly* and how the hell you keep it strong.

Ageing, running, and also pregnancy, thanks to the growing weight of a baby bedding in and making itself comfortable, can all have a considerable impact on our pelvic floor health. Imagine what happens when you combine the latter two (or in Anniki's case, all three).

Lisa once went to a postnatal exercise class where they warned against high-impact exercise like running while pregnant because of potential damage to the pelvic floor. They demo'd this by stretching out a sheet of clingfilm to represent the pelvic floor, and bouncing a round gym weight – to represent the baby – on top of it.

Everyone watching crossed their legs protectively as the weight stretched and warped its protective, sandwichy hammock. Imagine her horror when she later found postnatal exercise DVDs and classes which failed to mention the pelvic floor or the damage you could do with high-impact exercises while your body is in this fragile recovery period.

What about the sex angle, Hotbed?! We're not that interested in continence as a reading topic, to be honest …

When we say we want orgasm equality we *mean* it, and when we say it's not that difficult, we mean that too. And when we are asked what the single most important solution to closing the gap is, we say better pelvic floor awareness.

It's not immediately sexy. It is not immediately glamorous. It's a far cry from suggesting that you book a date night and wear hot knickers or go away for the weekend and put that 'Do not Disturb' sign on the door for forty-eight hours straight. It probably won't cause a Twitter storm or go viral or be an Instagram photo opportunity or make any headlines or get us invited to Buckingham Palace or have brands lining up to sponsor us or celebrities knocking down the door to talk about us at the UN … but we have concluded that the pelvic floor is so important to women's health, their self-esteem and their ability to orgasm, that looking after it is our number-one recommendation.

The pelvic floor is a muscle and like most muscles, it needs to be exercised. When it is toned and treated to regular workouts, it performs better: it allows greater blood flow to the pubic area, the nerves get more sensitive, and the stronger the sensation against your clitoris can be.

Some women have been known to orgasm simply from squeezing their pelvic floor muscles during exercise, sometimes known as a 'coregasm'. (On their way out from recording a podcast together at the Acast studio in Shoreditch, London, Lisa and the poet Hollie McNish once had quite a loud conversation about their experiences of coregasming.) Squeezing and releasing your pelvic floor during sex or masturbation (see p.268) is a known orgasm technique. If you are having sex with a male-bodied partner, it can feel great for them too, but warn them before you do it just in case you catch them off-guard.

If you are about to have a baby, doing your exercises will help protect the muscles against the pressure of the growing baby, and it is also thought that a strong pelvic floor, and an ability to do the 'release' part of the exercise (as outlined below), can help push the baby down the birth canal. And trust us, anything that makes birth easier is worth a punt.

A strong core also helps keep you standing straight and tall, giving you the posture of a ballerina even if you, like us, have as much grace as a recycling truck. Some people refer to it as an 'inner corset', keeping you zipped in and upright but, sadly, without the resultant mega cleavage. Last but not least, the more ripped the pelvic floor muscle is, the tighter and tauter your vagina will feel. This can be a great confidence boost as you get older or after you have had a baby.

All this, and protection against wetting or shitting your pants? Sounds like a good idea to us.

So why the silence, you may ask?

Like many topics which we tackle, in the pelvic floor health is simply not talked about enough and that vacuum makes space for shame and misinformation.

Women will head to the GP six weeks after giving birth, and very few of these GPs will ask about the pelvic floor, even fewer will glove up and check internally. Women's health physiotherapists exist but the NHS may only refer if there is severe pelvic floor dysfunction such as prolapse (when one of your internal organs starts slipping down into the vagina). If you have the wherewithal you can choose to go private, but it is expensive (£40–80 for one session).

Consequently, like Lisa in the story above, women put up with wetting themselves: either just a little bit every time they sneeze, or the whole kahuna when they step onto a trampoline. Having even a minor pelvic floor dysfunction makes your life the opposite of those 'woah, Bodyform' adverts showing women jumping around with a lust for life usually preserved for when Beyoncé headlines Glastonbury. It makes you self-conscious about sneezing, jumping, laughing and exercising. It makes sex painful. It can suck the joy out of your life.

And what do we do instead? We paper over the cracks with incontinence pads, laugh about it to trusted friends (while crossing our legs and clenching like mad), and decide that that is just what our life is now.

Many women suffer in silence, but we are here to tell you that it is not the only option. Any bit of accidental weeing is a sign of a problem and time to take action. As is any pain or discomfort when you pee or poop, or if you feel a heavy or dragging sensation in your vagina.

And just to be clear: although pelvic floor problems become more apparent after pregnancy and as we grow older and reach the menopause, there is still a risk of it happening at any age, and even the youngest, bounciest of women should still be doing exercises to look after their pelvic floor, not only for the sex benefits.

After her unfortunate nativity incident, here are some of the things that Lisa tried:

YOGA

I love yoga and the 'mulabandha' movement which is, essentially, a pelvic floor squeeze incorporated into yoga moves. It is integral to many practices, and is excellent for getting the pelvic floor back into shape. But I found that, unless you have private tuition, it's hard to find a class which will have this as a focus.

REBOUNDING

This is when you jump up and down on a teeny-tiny trampoline in a room full of happy, sweaty people all getting their groove on. Every time you bounce you give your pelvic floor a little workout, and the bonus is that they sometimes play old-school UK garage music.

The downside is that you need to do a bit of work on the pelvic floor *before* you start bouncing (and, ideally, go to the loo), because it can be a bit much for those defeated muscles otherwise, and piss stains on your Lycra is not a good look.

KEGEL BALLS

These are a bit sexy (they are a series of balls of different sizes and weights which you insert inside your vagina while you carry on with your day, giving the pelvic floor a workout with every step), so I tried to trick myself into thinking it was actually foreplay, not exercise. But, while a strong pelvic floor has massive advantages when it comes to getting your sex life back after kids, using the balls themselves is a bit fiddly and intimidating when you're not on form.

THE ELVIE

The elvie is a pelvic floor exerciser which connects via Bluetooth to an app on your phone. So, when you clench and squeeze, not only are you told whether or not you are doing it right, but you get to play cool little computer games while you do it. Imagine playing Tetris with your vagina and you are kind of there. I was so impressed and entertained by the idea that, for the first time in my life, I did the exercises as much as I was supposed to and, within a month, I could say 'so long, suckers' to those pantyliners. Sex stopped hurting too. It isn't cheap but the good news is that the elvie is about to be offered on the NHS. Result.

SOME OTHER WAYS TO RESTORE THE PELVIC FLOOR

SPEAK TO YOUR GP AND ASK FOR A REFERRAL TO A WOMEN'S HEALTH PHYSIO. If they can't make the referral, go to the Pelvic, Obstetric and Gynaecological Physiotherapy website (pogp.csp.org.uk) to find a local practitioner. If cost is an issue, call around to find the best deal, and explain that you can only afford one session so to fit in as much as they can in that time.

INCORPORATE PELVIC FLOOR EXERCISES INTO YOUR NORMAL ROUTINE. Remind yourself with Post-it notes with code words such as 'First Floor' or give yourself a cue such as 'every time I'm waiting at a red light, I will squeeze'.

Once you know how to do the exercises, incorporate them into everyday movement and gym moves or lifting heavy objects/children — not only does this make the actions easier, but it protects you at the same time.

DOWNLOAD THE 'SQUEEZY' APP, which guides you through the exercises and can be linked up with your physio, if you have one, so they can set you exercises.

PILATES AND BALLET BAR are also great exercises for your core, and the average teacher of these disciplines should be well versed in the importance of posture, alignment and how to incorporate the squeeze into the activity. If they don't mention it — ask them at the end of the class.

As ever, open up the conversation about this. Telling your doctor is one thing, but don't be afraid to tell your mum that you're retraining your pelvic floor, or to ask a friend who's just had a baby how her pelvic floor is. Women's health matters, and getting it taken seriously can start with a simple conversation.

If you have read this far without frantically clenching and releasing, we're surprised. But now let's take a moment to make sure we are doing pelvic floor exercises properly ...

HOW TO EXERCISE YOUR PELVIC FLOOR PROPERLY

By the Mummy Coach, AKA personal trainer and pelvic floor campaigner Elizabeth Davies.

First things first, a little disclaimer: pelvic floor exercises are most effective when individually tailored to the pelvic floor. This is the benefit of seeing a women's health physio who can assess what is right for you. The exercises described here are just a guide.

1.

Start by getting into good alignment. Stand in front of a mirror side-on with your feet hip-width apart. Find your neutral pelvis by tilting the pelvis through full range and stopping at the midway point. You don't want it sticking too far out but you don't want it completely tucked under, either.

2.

Next make sure that your ribcage is stacked over your pelvis, so that it isn't pointing up or pointing down. Create length through the spine as if someone has a strand of your hair and is pulling it to the ceiling, but don't jut the chest out in the process. Take a big roll back with the shoulders and let them fall. Tuck in your chin.

3.

Next you need to identify the correct muscles. Do this by imagining first that you are stopping the flow of urine; second that you are sucking a milkshake up a straw inside your vagina; and third that you are trying to stop a fart in a very important work meeting. Play around with this if you need to. You may find that the fart is really easy but the wee not so much, or vice versa.

4.

Once you've got the muscles, start with some slow contractions. Take an inhale into the ribs. Imagine the ribs opening up like an umbrella. Relax the pelvic floor, abs, inner thighs, bum and jaw. As you exhale through soft lips imagine you are simultaneously stopping the flow of wee, sucking a milkshake through the vagina and stopping a fart as you lift the whole of the pelvic floor. Continue to keep your abs, inner thighs, bum and jaw relaxed as you do this. Try to hold the contraction for ten seconds, but stop if you begin clenching any of the other muscles.

5.

Inhale and fully relax the pelvic floor (this is very important, because, as with any muscle, we need to train through full range by relaxing between contractions). Try to do ten repetitions of these slow contractions but with pelvic floor exercises, remember, it's quality very much over quantity.

6.

We also need to train the pelvic floor with fast contractions. Keep your abs, inner thighs, bum and jaw relaxed. Quickly lift the pelvic floor, keeping all of the other muscles unclenched and relaxed. Then slowly relax the whole of the pelvic floor. Try to do ten of repetitions of these fast contractions followed by a slow release, but heed the advice concerning quality not quantity, above. Breathe in a way that's comfortable for you throughout these exercises, remembering not to hold your breath at any point.

OK, Hotbed, we get the point. We're squeezing now and it's making us feel a bit horny to be quite honest ...

Our work here is done ...

Long-Term Lovers: the Reality

15

Flashback to a first date at Slug &
Lettuce, Westbourne Grove, 1998:

ANNIKI is sitting at a table
nervously smoking (yes, you could
still smoke in pubs back then. She
checks the door to see if her date
has walked in yet. She's wearing
a lot of make-up (this is before
foundation that matched your skin
tone and she has a mark where her
face starts and her neck ends.

She is wearing Buffalo platform
trainers that she's unable to walk
in. There is nothing to distract
her while she waits because
mobiles are only carried by
yuppies, and are the size of
toasters. She's waiting for a guy
that she likes. The last time
they met they were both drunk and
snogged for three hours.

She isn't sure what he looks like
but remembers that he smelt good
and wore a leather jacket.

PAUL walks in.

He is tall, wearing the selfsame
leather jacket. ANNIKI is pleased.
He looks like a less skeletal version of Richard Ashcroft.

                    PAUL
        [Smiling] Hey, how are you?

ANNIKI drops her matches all over
the floor and has to crawl under
the table to retrieve them. She
bumps her head on the underside of
the table. She thinks about
pulling PAUL under the table so
they can snog.

                    PAUL
      Are you OK? Do you want a drink?

ANNIKI continues to pick up
matches and mumbles that she'd
like a 'Smirnoff Mule'. She
manages to sit down and lights her
seventh cigarette. Her date is
more handsome than she remembered.
She feels funny inside. She
wonders what PAUL will be like in
bed. He isn't like anyone she's
met before. He has a strong
masculinity about him.

PAUL sits down and they stare at
one other, saying very little.

ANNIKI drops her matches for a second time. Their conversation is stilted but the music is loud and after four drinks they go outside and snog. This goes on for a LONG time.

ANNIKI suggests they go somewhere else but then realises she is being too keen. Instead they agree to see one another the following weekend.

ANNIKI is incredibly excited. She can't stop thinking about this man. He may just be the sexiest man alive. PAUL is also excited. He thinks she's cute but also the clumsiest person he's ever met.

Fast-forward to 2018, a front room in West London:

ANNIKI is lying on the sofa, in a pair of decrepit jogging bottoms and a sweatshirt.

She has no make-up on and her hair is in a top knot (with the faint whiff of the dry shampoo she's used four days on the trot). She's casually picking off the dried skin from her chapped lips while staring gormlessly at the TV.

PAUL is lying on the floor scrolling through his iPad. He's looking at Pringle socks on eBay.

ANNIKI
Is this the only thing that's on tonight?

PAUL
Huh? [he continues to scroll through the display of socks on his screen and doesn't look up]

ANNIKI
I fancy some crisps. Are there any of those Maple Syrup and Bacon ones?

She gets up, looks in the cupboard, then stares wearily at the kitchen clock. She might go to bed anyway. Her daughter will be up in five hours. She doesn't bother saying goodnight.

PAUL
Did you find the crisps? Did you?

There's no reply - just the whirr of the electric toothbrush upstairs as Anniki resolves to brush her teeth for at least two minutes tonight. She can't be bothered with cleaning her face so it can wait until morning.

Spot the difference between these two scenes? For a start, you'll note that the first one is *romantic*. It could be a scene from a romcom. It's hot with sexual anticipation. Anniki drops the matches because she's full of excitement. She can't wait to snog. She can't wait for the two of them to have sex. It's the rock-and-roll stage of the relationship. It's what Led Zeppelin, the Rolling Stones and all those other rock dinosaurs based their entire careers singing on.

The problem is we've been brought up on Disney films and romantic comedies. Usually the core focus of these films is *bagging the man*, and then living happily ever after. However, you've quite possibly grown up in a reality where many parents (including your own) are divorced. Perhaps your parents remarried. Perhaps you were privy to some of the relationship problems. Perhaps these relationships weren't always cast in a glorious light.

On the one hand, there's the romantic side – the side that believes relationships should last for ever and everything is hunky-dory. On the other, the real world, and the fact that so many relationships end in divorce (currently forty-two per cent of marriages in the UK end this way).

Those early days in a relationship are often syncopated with lots of snogging, sex (sometimes multiple times in the same night) and inappropriate thoughts that crop into our heads at all hours. It's an exhilarating time. We feel horny. We can't wait to see the other person.

Our universe becomes incredibly small — it's just about that one person, how that person makes us feel, and when we're going to see them again.

In short, it's heaven.

This can go on for quite some time but for the majority of us the excitement fades and real life kicks in.

We fart in front of each other for the first time.

We get slightly bored by something they've said and don't listen properly.

They get on our nerves a few times.

We notice they've got hair growing out of their ears.

They notice we have blackheads on our nose.

We cut our hair and they don't mention it.

They buy a new jacket and we don't notice.

We find ourselves eyeing up a man on the escalator and wondering what he looks like with no trousers on.

Oh, and then there's kids.

Nora Ephron, the late celebrated author and screen-writer, once said that when you have a baby 'you set off an explosion in your marriage'. And we're not talking a sexy explosion either. Everything is recalibrated and the baby becomes the centre of the universe (because it needs to be in order to survive).

Sometimes a lot of anger and tiredness is directed towards one another because the baby is too small a thing to blame. Add to this the impact of childbirth/Caesarean surgery on women's bodies, and the way they're made to feel about post-baby weight, and you can easily see how sex gets put on the back burner.

When *The Hotbed* did a survey into couples with kids we found that the clear majority (seventy-seven per cent) were unhappy with their sex lives. A whopping ninety-three per cent also said they'd like them to improve, and more than a quarter said that they couldn't talk openly and honestly about this issue.

That last statistic, the one where people feel they can't talk about their sex lives, is a telling one. Many of us sit in our relationships feeling isolated. We can't talk to our partners about what's going on. The issue itself feels huge and unwieldy. We also worry about chatting to friends about it (because they're probably having sex all over the place, right?).

Seeking help and fessing up to a rubbish/non-existent sex life makes us feel incredibly vulnerable. This is particularly true if the culture around you is a sexy one, where TV programmes and movies and books and celebrities all seem to be copping off with one another.

We expect an awful lot of our relationships these days, and they have to perform a myriad of different functions. There's the romantic angle, the sex angle, maybe the parenting angle, then there's the whole day-to-day-running-of-the-house/admin/drudge angle.

Relationships in real life don't just magically fix themselves. It is a dangerous myth that functional people shouldn't have to actively work on their relationships. Relationships require work. They require effort. They require prioritising. This is a drag as there are so many other things competing for our time and energy. It's easy to file the 'non-satisfying sex life thing' next to 'must clean out cat litter tray' and 'need to buy a new wok next time in Ikea'. A year passes. Then two, and meanwhile the 'non-satisfying sex life thing' has escalated and it's now way more important than the cat litter and wok.

Esther Perel, a celebrated relationship psychotherapist (check out her excellent podcast *Where Should We Begin?)* said in a recent interview:

> *People have known love forever but it has never existed in the same relationship where you have to have a family and obligations. And reconciling security and adventure, or love and desire, or connection and separateness, is not something you solve with Victoria's Secret.*

There are no simple answers. Switching from the domestic you to the sensual you *is* a challenge and flashing some saucy underpants or booking a table for two at Carluccio's is unlikely to cut it.

Some of the most common things we hear from our listeners and readers include:

> *I thought I was the only one going through this.*

> *I feel so lonely. I want to have sex more often but just don't know where to start.*

> *My friends would be aghast if they knew the truth – the fact that we haven't had sex in six months now. I mean it's terrible, right?*

> *I wish I knew what to do next. I feel paralysed and stuck in a rut when everyone else out there is getting on with their lives.*

One of the most googled phrases is 'sexless marriage'. A lot of people are in the same boat. However, if you turned on the TV then you might not believe this to be true. It's rare to see realistic depictions of sex in long-term relationships (although there have been some recent notable exceptions, including the BBC's *Wanderlust* and Channel 4's *Catastrophe*, both encouraging examples).

If you're in it for the long haul, then it's unrealistic to expect it to be perfect. Yes, there may be the odd friend who claims she does it three times a week but the truth is that, in most relationships, sex ebbs and flows. If you have kids then the baby phase is fraught and tiring. Sex is not a priority. That's OK. That's probably a time to file it for a while and not place unwarranted pressure on the relationship.

Whatever your situation, it's important to remember that you're not alone: there is help and you will get through this (if you want to, that is).

TURNING A NEGATIVE INTO A POSITIVE

All too often the long-term relationship can lack appeal. It's all about compromise. Comfy clothes. Boxsets watched with bleary eyes with one eye on the baby monitor. Scrolling through our screens late at night watching other couples on date nights and no doubt having amazing sex afterwards (when date nights are the last thing you need – who wants a weighty, rich dinner and then sex?).

So, as a first step, The Hotbed have reviewed some of the most common misconceptions about long-term relationships and sex. We've tried to give them a positive spin, some rebranding, so to speak.

See if any of them shake up your own prejudices ... Hopefully they'll help you see the picture in a more positive light.

Sex in long-term relationships is boring …

Is it boring? Does it *have* to be boring?

Think about the benefit(s) of sex with someone you know *really* well. For a start, you don't need to pretend you like something (you should never do this anyway but we fall into traps in those early days and don't always say what we want).

Flip that frown upside down and remember your partner knows your body better than anyone else out there and there's lots of potential for them to bring you to orgasm: a lot of bad sex is down to a *lack* of familiarity, the fact that we're not open about what we enjoy. In a long-term relationship this isn't the case (if it is, then it's about better communication — having the nerve to say what you want sex-wise). You can and should be candid, i.e. 'I like it when you touch my clitoris in that way, so please do some more of that.'

Another fact to remember is that desire is not always spontaneous. Dr Rosemary Basson, a clinical sex therapist, noticed that many of her female patients took a while to become aroused (and there's evidence that men feel this way too). Desire was felt in response to a specific stimulus, i.e. it's a myth that you suddenly get the urge to jump on your partner and make mad and furious love to him/her. Basson argues that sexual response is cyclical and desire isn't always the first step in the process (this goes against the famous Masters and Johnson research in the Sixties). What this means in practical terms is that foreplay, sexy talk, visual stimulation, physical stimulation, all these things create desire but, unlike in the movies, it's rare to be overcome by desire without any stimulus at all.

In series three of our podcast we talked to journalist and author Sali Hughes, who stressed the importance of the 'maintenance shag' – the shag that *needs* to happen. You probably both know it needs to happen, so you need to prioritise it. Interestingly, she talks about the warm-up – this might be a squeeze, a suggestive comment, a playful interaction. Again, it is rare in long-term relationships to be overcome by the kind of desire we feel in those heady early days: it's about being more overt and acknowledging that if you wait for the urge to come along, you may be waiting some time.

Sex in long-term relationships is not as good as sex in new relationships ...

Really? Think back to some of the sex you've had with people that you didn't know well. Was it good? Or was it awful? The latter, we bet. We've already described a few examples of bad sex – oftentimes it's when you don't know someone and are too embarrassed to say you don't like their form (e.g. 'Having sex through my thick tights isn't working for me right now').

If you think about it logically, sex in a long-term relationship has oodles of potential. You're older, you know what you want, you know one another. You are not dealing with someone who thinks shoving a fistful of fingers into your vagina while talking dirty is a turn-on (unless it is a turn on, horses for courses etc.)

It's liberating to realise that a long-term relationship can deliver a different kind of sex. Maybe even a more orgasmic kind of sex.

'THE VERY THOUGHT OF YOU HAS MY LEGS SPREAD APART LIKE AN EASEL WITH A CANVAS BEGGING FOR ART.'

Rupi Kaur

Sex in long-term relationships is hard work and I'm too tired ...

Yes, but wasn't sex in new relationships harder work? Think of the energy and time you put into those first dates. Think of all the anxieties you have forgotten about: did you worry about your hairy legs? Did you hold your tummy in and worry that your boobs were in an unflattering position? Perhaps you were mortified when you'd made a funny noise with your vagina and wanted the ground to open up and make swallow you?

Also, one more thing, if you're *super* tired then what's better than lying down? This more familiar, comfortable sex means you don't have to be Mrs Athletic-Sex-Crazy-Pants all night long. It can be lazy sex instead. The I-think-the-kids-are-asleep-so-let's-make-it-quick sex. Or the I-want-to-eat-my-M&S-Dine-in-For-Two-so-let's-get-on-with-it sex.

There's no need to pull out the big guns and be super elaborate. You live with this person. You don't have to worry that they'll never text you again.

Sex in long-term relationships is often replaced by arguing about how to load the dishwasher properly

Yes, this is a reality for many couples. It's no secret that nowadays we live busy lives with plenty of distractions (and even the cave-dwelling people of the past had domestic chores to feel resentful about). Esther Perel, in her book *Mating in Captivity: How to Keep Desire and Passion Alive in Long-Term Relationships*, claims that the increased domesticity of a long-term relationship — which she sees as a forced form of intimacy — is the death sentence for whatever erotic charge a couple may have once had between them. She writes:

> *When the impulse to share becomes obligatory, when personal boundaries are no longer respected, when only the shared space of togetherness is acknowledged and private*

space is denied, fusion replaces intimacy and possession co-opts love. It is also the kiss of death for sex. Deprived of enigma, intimacy becomes cruel when it excludes any possibility of discovery. Where there is nothing left to hide, there is nothing left to seek.

WAIT! BEFORE YOU BOOK A ONE-WAY SINGLE TICKET TO LAS VEGAS, THERE IS HOPE! In one of our *Hotbed* podcasts we talked with our resident expert, the brilliant Dr Karen Gurney, a clinical psychologist and psychosexologist at the Havelock Centre, about how tough it can feel to move from 'why didn't you take out the rubbish?' to 'I want to ravish you.'

The reality is that too many long-term relationships are mired in the ordinary and everyday versus the sexy and fun. Karen proffers some practical advice on how to increase 'sexual currency' in long-term relationships. She defines it thus:

Sexual currency is the things you'd only do with a partner rather than a friend. So, it could be kissing, flirting, sending a suggestive text, a sexy comment — the things that you probably used to do much more in the beginning of your relationship.

To increase sexual currency in your relationship, Dr Karen advises the following:

For a week try and ramp up these sexual gestures big and small — so for example, a

*lingering kiss before your other half leaves
for work or a sexy text when they're on the
bus home. Importantly these things provide '
stepping stones' from a domestic/drudge kind
of relationship to one that feels more sexual.
A relationship where you're more likely to
share sexual intimacy of some kind.'*

Don't use these stepping stones as a prelude to sex: yes,
sometimes sex might happen as a result of becoming a
more sexually charged couple but other times it's just
about changing the dynamic. What about just snogging
for the sake of it? What about tapping into those fun
things you did when your relationship was more about
sex and less about bingeing on boxsets?

In this context the *amount* of sex you're having each
week becomes less of an issue. Instead you're focusing
on the small things that help you connect sexually.
It's a commitment between the two of you that you
seriously want to shift the dynamic from one of
critique/boredom/annoyance to something closer to
what you had at the start. It's also a great technique if
you've just had a baby, or are going through the menopause and don't actually want to have penetrative sex
for a while, but also don't want to feel like a dishcloth
that's been left out to dry either.

In essence, all long-term relationships benefit from a
boost of sexual currency once in a while. And remember,
the initial stepping stones might be quite small —

a pinch of the bum, a compliment — it's not about lungeing at your partner without warning (though that can work too if the timing feels right).

MAKE TIME FOR SEX

There are times when sex isn't simply a matter of feeling a bit rusty or getting back on the bicycle. This is when it's important to seek help. If you've been through a long sex drought (and you know what *feels long* for you), we recommend some form of counselling.

You can't be expected to sort it all out on your own and sometimes taking that first step towards seeking help shows your partner a) just how much you value them and want the two of you to stick together, and b) how you're not going to put the whole sex thing on the back burner for ever and ever.

Sometimes a lack of sex is symptomatic of wider relationship issues. Simmering resentments, hurt feelings, an affair, old issues coming to the fore — these things often are best tackled in a safe and trusted environment.

Perhaps a medical issue needs to be addressed. Do you have a male-bodied partner who is experiencing erectile dysfunction and could this be why they are putting sex off? In this case, the GP is probably the best port of call.

If you're approaching menopause (see our chapter on Growing Old Disgracefully, p.293), you may be in need of lubrication (we're a fan of lube whatever your age), a vaginal mousse or moisturiser, or perhaps you're suffering with lower libido. Again, the GP is your first port of call, but there are lots of online resources (see p.347).

SOME SUGGESTIONS FOR
COUNSELLING SERVICES TO TRY

RELATE is a tried-and-tested organisation whose relationship counsellors will help you navigate rocky patches and get to the bottom of the core issues in your relationship. **www.relate.org.uk**

THE HAVELOCK CLINIC offers couples counselling and therapy with a particular focus on sex problems. It's also where our marvellous Dr Karen Gurney resides. **www.thehavelockclinic.com**

THE NHS: talk to your GP about counselling services offered in your area. The NHS website also provides a breakdown of local contact details. **www.nhs.uk**

It's useful to remember the adage 'Rome wasn't built in a day'. Repairing a crappy sex life won't happen overnight either. It's about commitment. It's about actually caring whether sex happens or not. It's sometimes about switching off the TV, and just doing it (and not thinking about it too much).

DO YOU HAVE THE SEX LIFE YOU WANT?

700 responses

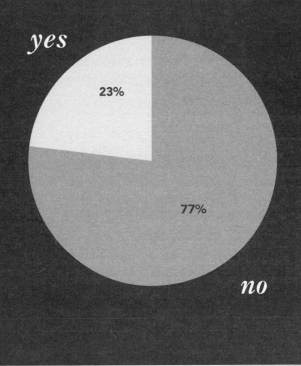

yes

23%

77%

no

This was from a survey about sex after kids, which also returned a 'yes' result of 93% to the question 'Would you like to improve your sex life?'

Growing Old Disgracefully

16

ANNIKI

I have a confession to make.

I'm old.

Not so old that I'm in the old-lady home. Or need assistance crossing the road. I'm forty-five. That makes me half way, or well over half way, to the end.

It also has other implications (for me anyway), including:

- *Men ignore me unless they're pushing seventy-five.*

- *I wake each morning and have to do a full body scan to work out which piece of my anatomy will be giving me jip all day.*

- *I can't dance in a club for fear of a young person posting a video up on their Snapchat entitled 'Mum dancing. Lol.'*

- *I develop crushes that aren't dissimilar to the crushes I had when I was a teenager (except now they make me feel like Vic Reeves in* Shooting Stars *when he used to rub his knees in a lascivious way whenever a pretty female celebrity was around).*

- *My sex drive is either very high (see above), very low (would rather watch TV but could be persuaded at a push) or non-existent (sex is too much like hard work, pass the biscuits).*

- *People constantly talk to me about Helen Mirren and remind me how 'fabulous she is for her age', even though she is in her seventies and I am not.*

One of the toughest things has been the fact that I've become invisible. I was never Britney Spears but, in my youth, I usually got at least a couple of builders yelling inappropriate comments as I walked past. I even got wolf-whistles when I was hungover and looked like shit. I'd also get men leaning out of white vans as they careered round corners shouting 'CHEER UP, LOVE! IT MIGHT NEVER HAPPEN.' And, on one memorable occasion, 'I want to stick my face in yer growler!'

Those heady days have passed.

Now when I pass a building site, I hear nothing but the tinkling of an old piece of rope tapping against a scaffolding pole. Maybe someone singing Rita Ora in the wrong key as he eats his lunch.

Closer to home, I have to rely on my trusty Instagram mates to blow the wind up my arse with 'Looking good, babes!' every time I post a selfie, and my partner is more likely to grunt something about the TV licence than to whisper sweet nothings into my ear. I bet Helen Mirren doesn't have to put up with that.

Compliments are important. They cost nothing and, provided they're coming from the person you want them to come from, they make us feel sexy. My building-site scenario might be something worthy of Laura Bates's Everyday Sexism project but, in a relationship or happy sexual encounter, compliments make us feel appreciated and safe which, in turn, help us to bring down our defence barriers and achieve an orgasm. They remind us that we are attractive to the person we are attracted to (not just from a 'looks' perspective), which leads potentially to better, more satisfying sex.

But does old age mean never being complimented again? If it does, then what I'd really like to do is invent a sexual self-esteem boosting robot that issued flattering comments at regular intervals (feel free to contact us if you're in Silicon Valley with oodles of dosh). Let's call the robot Alex (after the lovely actor Alexander Skarsgård). When you woke up, he'd say something like, 'Damn, you look mighty fine, woman.' When you stepped out the shower, he'd quip, 'Praise the Lord, you're a glorious woman with a body made for sin', and so on. (Alex's tone seems to be a bit Baptist preacher from the Deep South, but you get my gist.)

Oh, and one last thing, just so it's clear … I'm probably never going to be like Helen Mirren, OK?

Ageing = fewer compliments + being put in the same camp as Helen Mirren even though most women do not age like her = not a very sexy time for Anniki. So, no wonder she's a bit over sensitive on the subject of her age.

Because it's all very well holding up Dame Helen as an example of growing old gracefully — we love her, we really do — but Helen Mirren, and other glamorous older celebrities in her ilk, are often applauded for looking as they do *despite* being in their seventies, rather than *because* they are in their seventies. It's a subtle but important difference. And including Helen Mirren, or Twiggy, or Susan Sarandon, for example, in an ad campaign or magazine spread as a nod to age-diversity doesn't really make life any easier for the rest of us.

Those dames aside, many women in the public eye simply don't age and don't tell us why. We've lost count of the celebrity profiles where female actresses in their forties, fifties and sixties have declared how happy they are to be older, how they feel more confident, more sexual, and so on, and so far, so encouraging. Next to this feature, however, is usually a photo of this woman looking as if she is in her twenties, dancing about like she's never experienced a creaking joint, or hairy upper lip and chin, in her life.

What's all that about? How is it possible to look like this at fifty-five?

Perhaps these women are of that rare breed that is naturally graced with fantastic genes and enduring youthfulness, and fair play to them. We wish we had their genes! More likely, though, we suspect that said 'celeb' has perhaps forgotten to mention in the interview that they've had a little help from a cosmetic surgeon.

Or even if that's not the case, they have probably spent a lifetime and small fortune on personal trainers and diet plans, *or* had a ton-load of non-invasive cosmetic procedures, *or* they simply had a very good make-up artist and photo editor.

To the rest of us, though, with our saggy faces and stretch marks and turkey-droop elbows (why does elbow skin continue to grow so it hangs lower than our forearms?), it doesn't seem fair. It can be pretty dis-piriting at times too.

As women, we're raised to believe that our currency — sexual and otherwise — is based on our outward appear-ance. Our glossy hair, white teeth and perfect features are dissected and evaluated (there's a 'golden ratio' that relates to the ideal vertical and horizontal dimensions of the human face). Our boobs should be springy; our butts high, tight and round; our thighs muscular, but not so much that they look masculine.

The 'ideal' body shape has changed over the decades: from the athletic 'flapper' look of the Twenties, to the curve-o-rama boobs'n'booty look defined by the Kardashian clan, but at any one time the definition of perfect is narrow, and it is always youthful. There aren't very many big ad campaigns using older women (with the rare exceptions, in fact, you usually only see women over fifty selling stand-up baths and stair-lifts ...).

Fortune favours the fair-of-face and toned-of-body, and it has a very real economic impact on women as they get older: fading looks = fading job prospects, fewer promotions, and having to wait the longest to be served at the bar. Alas, we live in a value-based society, and older women too often can feel that they are seen as having little or no value, or rather they cease to be seen at all.

Ageing can make us feel like we're losing our sex appeal and we struggle to see anyone out there that reflects our life stage. Sex is all tied up with self-confidence and the physical effects of ageing take their toll on that confidence.

(**Full disclosure alert**: Anniki has tried Botox and counts herself in the Botox-faced camp. She hasn't had it for quite a while, though, and she's coming clean right now. And did it make her feel any better? No, it didn't. Plus, orgasms are cheaper and quite effective at giving you a nice, youthful glow.)

Hey, Hotbed! Give us some positive vibes here, mate!

Whatever the dominant culture feeds us about ageing, a lot of women really do feel better and some say that they feel more sexy, and appreciate their looks more, as they age.

As celebrated journalist India Knight writes in *In Your Prime*, her book about middle age:

> *I feel exactly like I've always felt, except better, in so many respects: more confident,*

> *more self-assured, more unwilling to take any*
> *crap. I mind more about the things that are*
> *important to me, and I've stopped minding*
> *about the things that aren't.*

India Knight's book spoke to us because it describes someone who is happy in their own skin. In some ways, it can be a relief to no longer feel under so much pressure to conform to some supposed ideal of perfect, or sexy, or to feel like a mere object of the male gaze.

Indeed, if you found those unsolicited comments and compliments on our appearance to be more like minor aggressions (and many times they are), and if you want to be able not to worry about what people think, old age can be a respite. With age can come clarity and the confidence to choose how to play your own game. Dress to impress when you want to, not because you feel you always *have to* look a certain part. And if you feel like cutting loose in a comfy fleece and elasticated track pants, rock on. This is how most men walk through life, after all.

Whoopi Goldberg, actress and presenter of *The View* (the American equivalent of *Loose Women* and we bloody love it) has tried marriage three times and, in the wisdom of her years, has the confidence to conclude that monogamy is not for her. She has written all about it in her book, *If Someone Says 'You Complete Me'* *— Run!*

And then there's the outspoken, seldom apologetic broadcaster Janet Street-Porter (at The Hotbed we call her simply Big J). In her book *Life's Too F***ing Short* (great title) Big J writes:

> *Life's too fucking short to get depressed about being forty-something ... to talk to people who are boring, to spend it [time] in the same dreary job ... to have a set of rules you can't live up to.*

We added a few things to this list:

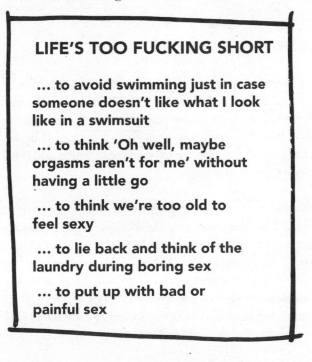

LIFE'S TOO FUCKING SHORT

... to avoid swimming just in case someone doesn't like what I look like in a swimsuit

... to think 'Oh well, maybe orgasms aren't for me' without having a little go

... to think we're too old to feel sexy

... to lie back and think of the laundry during boring sex

... to put up with bad or painful sex

Once we accept that the marks of age come to us all sooner or later, growing older can be extremely liberating. We're less willing to tolerate bullshit. We can cut to the chase, question dominant narratives (i.e. the male gaze) and be more assertive in terms of what we want. Sex in our fifties, sixties and beyond can potentially be the best of our lives. Jane Fonda talking about sex in later life said, 'first of all, we're braver — what the heck to we have to lose? So my skin sags — so does his.' Fonda also pointed out that the depiction of older age and sexuality was improving (*Grace and Frankie*, the Netflix show she stars in, is a good example of this).

Older people can be sexy, and older sex can be sexy.

In theory, by the time we start saying, 'Ooh, nice to sit down', and no longer have to pretend we like music festivals, we should also know our own bodies inside out. We know what we want from a partner. The key thing is making sure we express these truths and don't keep them bottled up.

It's also worth remembering the era that you were born into. The older you are, the potentially less sexually expressive culture you were born into. You may have more hang-ups and prejudices because the way you were schooled was restrictive and rigid in its definition of sexuality. One of the first challenges is asking yourself, 'Do I believe these things I learnt back then? Or is it time to cast them off and get on with my life?'

There is another key truth about ageing. You will never be as young as you are in this moment. Journalist

Sophie Heawood has written about the famous Nora Ephron quote on ageing (Ephron basically says she wished she'd worn a bikini when she was twenty-six instead of covering up):

> *We'll probably be livid with ourselves for not wearing a bikini when we looked perfectly lovely at forty. And so, it goes on. We keep saying we should have done things when we were younger – why not do them now?*

SEX AND AGEING IN POPULAR CULTURE

We need to change the narrative around older people having sex in popular culture, because if we feel uneasy about seeing older people having sex then is it any surprise that our personal relationship with ageing is so ambivalent (and downright negative)?

As with body positivity, being age-positive is important, and the truth is that we see very little out there at present to normalise and celebrate the simple fact that older people have sex – and orgasms – too. All too often, sex scenes and the subject of sex once anyone is over sixty is played for laughs: as it's deemed too unspeakable or embarrassing to be mentioned or shown without eliciting a nervous snigger, and/or cries of 'Gross!'. In 2004, for example, when Anne Reid starred alongside Daniel Craig in a film called *The*

Mother, about a woman having sex with her daughter's boyfriend, a man half her age, there was an outcry because audiences just weren't used to seeing older women as sexually desirable, not least to younger men.

A happy exception to this rule is Barbra Streisand's role in *Meet the Fockers*. It's a brilliantly funny film and Streisand is glorious in it. For those who haven't had the joy of watching it, we can't recommend it enough. Barbra (or, as we call her at The Hotbed, Big B) plays Mrs Focker senior, Ben Stiller's onscreen mum, a sex therapist who specialises in the older age range. In one scene we see her and Mr Focker senior, her husband (played by Dustin Hoffman), indulge in some funny, sexy role play. Later in the film, Ben Stiller winds up in jail and the judge turns out to be one of her clients. He's so grateful for all she taught him about how to please his wife that he lets him off scot-free. She's a fantastic character and we love that she is so matter of fact about sex, and isn't afraid of talking about it to the other, stiffer characters, or indulging in lots of action herself. She's our ideal vision of our older, still sexy, fun and liberated selves. We say we should all vow to Be More Barbra.

We need a mind-shift and to see more positive affirmations of the joy of sex regardless of our age. So, when a film or TV series depicts older people having sex or masturbating in a way which isn't 'Ew, gross, that's like seeing my parents at it', tweet about it and try to get their ratings up. Life's too short not to celebrate things like this.

THE TRUTH ABOUT SEX AND AGE

What *does* getting older mean for our sex lives? The bad news first — our bodies are actually ageing and for women this means the menopause, which can play havoc with the sex side of things. The menopause is different for every woman and you may not experience all or any of these, but common symptoms can include vaginal dryness, discomfort during sex, hot flushes (not related to fantasising about Ryan Gosling), low mood, anxiety, extreme fatigue, low motivation, reduced sex drive, night sweats and more hot flushes.

So, first off, the menopause is something we need to face up to, and talk about. See your GP and discuss treatment options and ways to cope with symptoms. Don't suffer in silence or feel too embarrassed to share your experience and let your partner — if you have one — know how you are feeling. It won't go away just because Jennifer Lopez is dating a man half her age and still looks the same as she did in the 'Jenny from the Block' video.

Happily, there's now a movement developing and more and more women are talking openly about their menopause — from Meg Matthews and her website www. megsmenopause.com, to former Liberty X singer and author of *Hot Flush: Motherhood, Menopause and Me,* Michelle Heaton, who went through early menopause, to broadcaster Kirsty Wark's documentary *The Menopause and Me*. There's also Andrea McClean's book *Confessions of a Menopausal Woman*, which gives an honest and forthright account. All these personal narratives can only be a good thing.

There are lots of treatments that can help counteract some of the key side effects, but it's worth knowing that sex might not be top of the agenda for some time and that's OK too.

As previously mentioned, we strongly urge you to see your GP and talk openly about any concerns that might be causing a problem with your sex life or your ability to orgasm. We also feel that the medical profession could take the lead more and take proactive measures to help and inform women (and men) as they get older. An American study found that half of people aged between fifty-seven and eighty-five, who were sexually active, reported at least one sex-related health problem, and yet very few of these people had discussed the issue with a doctor. We understand that there are extreme time pressures and limited resources, but would it be so difficult for health professionals to ask patients about their sex life as part of a routine appointment? Is it inappropriate? Taboo? How would you feel if your doctor raised the subject with you? It could be that it's a relief to share a problem such as vaginal dryness and to know that lubricants may be available to you on prescription and, if they're not, they don't cost a lot of money. Any underlying health issues could be preventative too, as sexual problems can be a sign of an underlying issue such as infection or more serious illness — it goes without saying too that getting help sooner rather than later is always a good thing.

We've said it before, but it's worth reiterating that, of course, the day-to-day experience of ageing, the menopause and sex will be different for all of us. Expectations and what is 'normal' or desirable can vary wildly from person to person: standard, rigid definitions of life stage no longer exist. As Miranda Sawyer points out in *Out of Time*, her fab book about age and hitting forty, we don't all slip into our cardies and sip Bailey's in front of *The Two Ronnies* any more:

> *All this stuff is made doubly, triply confusing by the fact that, traditionally, at forty-five you would almost certainly have been a grandmother. Today, you may be the mother of a toddler. Or be both a grandmother and have a young child of your own.*

This can be both liberating and confusing: 'It's OK to wear this Topshop dress but if I drink two litres of Prosecco and try to snog my friend's son then it's not. I'm excited about buying a fleece floor-length nightie from Debenhams but feel like I should be booking an all-girls' holiday to Ibiza instead.'

The same applies on the sex front — you may be coming out of a divorce and immersing yourself in online dating and one-night stands. Or you might be in a twenty-year relationship and facing the challenges of keeping that fresh. You may be googling female equivalents of Viagra and begging your American friends to bring you over some Flibanserin next time they visit (although, the jury is still out on this one, some studies show any benefits of this are outweighed by horrible side effects. Bummer). Getting older no longer means one set of rules in and out of the bedroom.

'AT SEVENTY-FOUR, I HAVE NEVER HAD SUCH A FULFILLING SEX LIFE. WHEN I WAS YOUNG I HAD SO MANY INHIBITIONS – I DIDN'T KNOW WHAT I DESIRED.'

Jane Fonda

REASONS TO BE CHEERFUL ABOUT SEX IN YOUR FORTIES, FIFTIES, SIXTIES AND BEYOND

While men experience fewer orgasms as they age, women get more orgasmic as they get older. *Let us repeat that: Women get more orgasmic as they age.* One study, which tracked 800 women over a number of years, found that more than half of women aged eighty and above experienced 'sexual satisfaction always or almost always'. We'll take that, thank you very much …

… What's more, orgasms have lots of beautifying, youth-giving benefits (and are cheaper and less risky than injectables).

Some believe that the clitoris gets bigger as a woman ages. Some scientists say this is a load of baloney and, even if it is true, size isn't related to pleasure anyway, but still.

Remember those teenage days when you endured terrible sex because you were too scared to say you weren't enjoying that painfully enthusiastic fingering? Well, they're over. Ding-dong. Now is not the time to put up with any crap: you can do exactly what you want. Screw the idea of taking up watercolours. Why not write up a list of things you'd like to do sex-wise? Fancy some role play? Want to watch porn with your partner? Masturbate while you're watching *MasterChef*? Your time on this planet is finite. Get on with it!

TIPS ON WEATHERING WORRIES ABOUT GETTING OLDER

Remember you will never be as young as you are in this moment reading this (Anniki's Mum has this postcard in her front room and it always lifts her out of the ageing dumps)

Try using lube (see our Lube Chart on p.77)

When reading profiles of older actresses and celebrities, pay no attention to the way they look. They did not get that face from vaginal steaming and quinoa muffins for breakfast. If it makes you feel better, colour in their teeth with biro

Don't feel guilty about crushes

Fantasies keep the blood pumping around

When clambering into your swimsuit/ getting undressed/seducing someone, repeat the phrase: 'What would Janet Street-Porter do?' Remember her motto: **LIFE'S TOO FUCKING SHORT**

On a serious note: if you are going through the menopause then make sure you get the medical help and advice you need (no amount of bucket lists or positive thinking will help if you're suffering serious side effects).

We live in crazy, age-confusing, turbulent times. Go forth. Explore. Have fun. Challenge the ageist trolls. And remember, on your deathbed you'll never regret the fact that you had too many orgasms.

WOULD YOU LIKE TO HAVE MORE ORGASMS?

1,217 responses

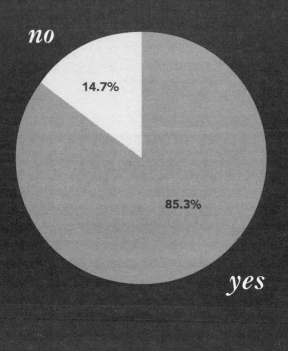

no

14.7%

85.3%

yes

Choice comments here are 'It's hard for women to break free of social stigmas and be open about wanting to orgasm', 'If I filled this in when I was 21 my answers would have been completely different. I'm glad I never gave up hope!' and 'Can you ever have too many?!'

The Future of Sex: Where Do We Go from Here?

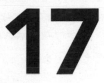

ANNIKI AND LISA

LISA: *So, we've covered a lot of ground, right? I mean, some might say we've covered TOO much.*

ANNIKI: *Well, you do go on a bit sometimes.*

LISA: *And you've got your head stuck in the Nineties and can't stop talking about Michael Hutchence despite the fact that he died more than twenty years ago now.*

ANNIKI: *Don't remind me ...*

LISA: *Anyway, this final chapter is supposed to be all about the future of sex: where we're headed; whether the orgasm gap will become a thing of the past; whether* *we can go forth and embrace our bodies, our age, our dodgy pelvic floor muscles, and create the sex lives we deserve.*

ANNIKI: *That was very arousing, what you just said there.*

LISA: *Well, I hope our readers feel the same way.*

ANNIKI: *The thing is, I'm often depressed when I think about the future.*

LISA: *Why? Is it because you're of an age considered no-longer-fuckable by the media?*

ANNIKI: *No, not just that … for a start, the stats show that people are having less sex, more relationships are failing, and we've not even talked about the whole technology thing. I mean, are we even going to have sex with* real people *in the future? Or will we be having it off with virtual avatars?*

LISA: *Here we go — 'I don't like this new-fangled tech stuff. I like the old-fashioned sex toys like you got in* Sex and the City. *At the turn of the last century when I came of age, we just had candles and bed posts to make do with … yadda yadda.'*

ANNIKI: *Hey, didn't you read the chapter about ageing? It's a positive thing — we can be old and relevant. I'm officially embracing my age like (ahem ... a younger) Helen Mirren. I might even start wearing my glasses in public. And dying my hair pink. Maybe I'll finally open that packet of lube I bought at our live podcast recording.*

LISA: *Go for it, mate. I'm actually positive about the future. It's going to bring new challenges and new opportunities. Good and bad. And if we don't believe the future will hold more orgasms for all, then who the hell does? And why am I talking in a way which only works when written down like a script of a fake conversation?*

Newspaper headlines tell us that we're getting less sex, being less intimate, feeling lonelier and, on top of that, suffering more stress, anxiety and mental illness. As we've outlined in this book, there are lots of negative stories around sex and the suppression of female sexuality specifically, but *we* must rewrite our stories and challenge the patriarchy ourselves.

It may sound a bit cheesy but we like this quote from Eleanor Roosevelt:

> *The future belongs to those who believe in the beauty of their dreams.*

And, in the (shamelessly appropriated to suit our own argument and topic) words of writer Arundhati Roy,

> *Another world is not only possible, she is on her way. On a quiet day, I can hear her breathing.*

So, if you find traditional porn depressing and reductive — vote with your eyes. Watch Erika Lust and some feminist porn instead. In an era when 'eyeball time' represents serious cash, choosing what to watch and what to kick to the kerb is important.

And if you're fed up of never having an orgasm, of rarely having an orgasm, then what are you going to do? We hope this book has convinced you that more orgasms are in your power, and has given you some advice on the physical and mental barriers which may have got in your way. But the next step is yours.

We can't physically come around to your house and give you an orgasm (we just don't have the woman power as there's only two of us) but we can remind you not to push it to one side and to make it a priority (if you want to, we're not 'orgasm bullies' either — although wouldn't that be a modern problem?).

We hope that this book might spark some conversations too. And some laughs. One thing we've learnt at The Hotbed is that once you start sharing and talking about sex, the more addictive it becomes, the more normalised, the more confident we feel, the more likely to prioritise sex above boxsets — all that good stuff and so much more.

Hey, Hotbed, you're making the future sound like a Hallmark Christmas card, but in the future won't we all be having sex with robots rather than with one another?

Tech can be an isolating force or it can be a force for good. It's complicated. If we use the analogy of Instagram, social media can bring people together, create deeper connections and help share experiences. It can also be a lonely, sad thing that makes you feel that you're missing out, which makes you depressed, and therefore less likely to engage in the world and with the people around you.

And yes, some people are choosing sex dolls and robots over real people.

For example, there are now people who choose to cohabit with sex dolls rather than with human partners. In a 2013 interview with the *Atlantic*, forty-year-old 'Davecat' explained why he'd chosen to live with 'Sidore' and 'Elena' versus pursuing human relationships — 'They [the dolls] don't possess any of the unpleasant qualities that organic, flesh and blood humans have. A synthetic will never lie to you, cheat on you, criticise you, or be otherwise disagreeable.'

We won't judge anybody's sexual choices (if they don't hurt anyone and are consensual), but the idea that you can dispatch with the mess and chaos of human relationships doesn't fill us with joy. Yes, humans are irritating and pick their feet on the sofa — but do we really want to trade them in for robots that (or should we say 'who'?) sit passively and are always receptive to our needs?

There are also people who are watching so much porn that it's depressing them or giving them unrealistic expectations of what sex is actually like. We need to talk about this stuff and stay open to what's happening. Information is power, right?

But enough scaremongering. Let's look at the exciting things, the tech that might be useful, things that create a sense of intimacy and help build relationships (versus replacing them entirely).

NEW TECH THAT CAN BRING COUPLES TOGETHER

Imagine you have a job which requires you to travel a lot. And, if you have a partner, the opportunities to get jiggy are limited. There's tech now which allows you to use a vibrator with pulses that can be controlled remotely by your partner via an app. Combine that with a video call, and it's more fun than room service or a drink by yourself in the bar.

Stephanie Alys is the former co-founder and Chief Pleasure Officer of MysteryVibe, a tech-enabled sex toy company. She gave a thought-provoking TED Talk called 'Why You Should Be Excited About the Future of Sex'. Alys outlines why technology isn't the thing we should fear, but rather the *way* we use it. She cites the example of virtual reality: what if we truly opened our minds and started to interrogate what we wanted in a virtual world of our choosing? Would we choose a man as a partner? Would we choose to be male or female? What about our body type? What about location? What if we could create a sexual scenario without being held back by patriarchal norms and expectations?

Tech might free us up, to feel more positive about our bodies, to try new things, not feel tied to narrow, stereo-typical, masculine definitions of pleasure. That sounds quite liberating, right?

SEX IS ALWAYS CHANGING AND SO THE WAY WE GET PLEASURE WILL CHANGE TOO ...

The first vibrator was invented in 1883, but before that there were candles, bananas, pieces of wood ... you name it. Sex tools have become more sophisti-cated, more customisable and more effective, and a truly mind-boggling plethora of gadgets and gizmos is now available to choose from. There might just be something that helps pep things up, and makes sex more exciting again. The Ole is a female sex toy which uses artificial intelligence to create orgasm-heavy vibes. It hit the headlines when it won a prize for innovation at a tech convention, only for the prize to be promptly revoked due to its 'vulgar' nature, which some thought was because it was a female sex toy (the same conference hosted a room of virtual reality porn for heterosexual men and this passed without comment). But there is definitely more outlandish gear on its way: just let your mind wander as you ponder on the possibilities.

Let's say this time, it's your partner who is away for work. He/she is sitting in a Travelodge, has just eaten a cheese and pickle sandwich from Boots and is feeling lonesome. Meanwhile you've managed to sort your laundry out, the rest of the household is asleep/out and you can't face another episode of *The Real Housewives of Cheshire* ... so, you and your partner reach for your virtual reality devices.

You climb into a suit which has hundreds of sensors built into it that stimulate different parts of your body. You engage in some chat about what kind of mood you're in tonight and then finally opt for the 'Dave Grohl' scenario from your preferred list of options. You choose a Malibu beach house with a perfect view of the sea. You opt to be female but love the idea of having butterfly wings so you can fly around the beach house. Your partner decides they want to be an alien/Dave Grohl hybrid instead. Let's face it, this experience is either going to be incredible or funny.

As couples, we must evolve to survive. If we keep doing the same things, at the same time, in the same context, then it's only ever going to breed boredom and fatigue.

There will also be some strange moral dilemmas. Like rethinking what fidelity means. Say you create a sex avatar that looks like a celebrity. Does that mean you've been unfaithful to your partner? And how do you think that celebrity feels? These complex dynamics will be something we'll have to navigate as the technology becomes more accessible.

TIPS FOR NAVIGATING FUTURE NEW TECH

Does the tech or gadget make you feel good? If you feel bad and out of kilter afterwards (and it's not just your typical sex-guilt that you get because you were raised Catholic), why do you think that is? What facet makes you uneasy? Is it the tech itself or the way you're using it or something else entirely?

Does it enhance your relationship with your other half? Does it feel like an avoidance strategy or is there a way to bring it into your lives so you can explore the potential together?

Does it liberate you to try things that you've always wanted to try? Or do you still find yourself conforming to certain sexual clichés? (Remember, not all of us hanker after BDSM scenarios where we're dressed in latex – it's not about feeling pressured to try extreme scenarios if they scare the Bejesus out of you)

So, it's not cut-and-dried then, is it, Hotbed?

If technology can offer up more orgasms then that's a good thing. Arguably, however, some of this new tech amplifies the negative sides of patriarchy, notably the sex dolls that look like porn stars, and virtual porn scenarios where women are dominated and ultimately exploited. This is no small thing. Commercial objectives will prevail (versus companies thinking about what's good for us, what will help us live better lives).

BUT ... the future doesn't have to be as awful as we think it might be. Let's remember that the way we se technology is our choice. We can control how we use these things and the role they could play in our lives: to connect, to empower, to enrich. *We* decide.

Technology that gives women more orgasms, opens people up to experiences they might not have had ... well, that's a step in the right direction. There are also new ways for couples to break out of sex droughts, play out different roles, and inject more fun and energy into their sex lives. The key question we need to ask ourselves will be, 'Does this tech *enhance* my relationship or does it just create more avoidance/isolation?'

Our sexual future is in our sweaty hands. We can put up with bad sex, never ask for cunnilingus, feel stale in our relationships, mournful for the past *or* we can open up the conversations.

We can ask for what we want. We can stop putting it off. We can challenge the status quo.

So yes, there are plenty of reasons to be positive about sex in the future. We've come a long way. It's up to us how we shape the next bit ...

AFTERWORD

We hope you have enjoyed reading our book, and that it has been useful, made you think, given you confidence, made you feel less alone, and helped to start a conversation, and to establish a new starting point for change.

We really hope so. And we hope you'll get in touch because we would love to hear from you and know your thoughts.

You are a goddess.

Please find us **@thehotbedcollective** on Instagram, or on our website **thehotbedcollective.com**.

REFERENCES

INTRODUCTION

13 *female desire is extremely responsive:* Catherine Coulson and Tessa Crowley, 'Current thoughts on psychosexual disorders in women', *The Obstetrician and Gynaecologist*, 9(4) (2007), pp. 217–22.

16 *Laughter also releases feel-good endorphins:* Sandra Manninen et al., 'Social laughter triggers endogenous opioid release in humans', *Journal of Neuroscience*, 37(25) (2017), pp. 6125–31.

18 *the good news is that most cases of anorgasmia are treatable:* Margaret M. Redelman, 'A general look at female orgasm and anorgasmia', *Sexual Health*, 3(3) (2006), pp. 143–53.

CHAPTER 1: WHAT EXACTLY IS AN ORGASM?

26 *a female orgasm is generally accepted to include:* 'What is an orgasm?', NHS website, www.nhs.uk/common-health-questions/sexual-health/what-is-an-orgasm/; Roy J. Levin, 'The pharmacology of the human female orgasm: its biological and physiological backgrounds', *Pharmacology Biochemistry and Behavior*, 121 (2014), pp. 62–70.

26 *Orgasms in women are a combination:* E. Emhardt, J. Siegel and L. Hoffman, 'Anatomic variation and orgasm: could variations in anatomy explain differences in orgasmic success?', *Clinical Anatomy*, 29(5) (2016), pp. 665–72.

26 *if you don't reach orgasm during vaginal intercourse alone:* Elizabeth Lloyd, *The Case of the Female Orgasm: Bias in the Science of Evolution* (Harvard University Press, 2005).

33 *female sexual satisfaction can have the following results:* Rachel Burge, 'Seven Amazing Health Benefits of Orgasms', AOL, 15 December 2016, www.aol.co.uk/living/2016/09/15/orgasms-sex-health-benefits/.

34 *The picture becomes more troubling:* John H. Frederick, Justin Garcia and Elisabeth Lloyd, 'Differences in orgasm frequency among gay, lesbian, bisexual, and heterosexual men and women in a US national sample', *Archives of Sexual Behavior*, 47(1) (2017), pp. 273–88.

34 *A Public Health England (PHE) survey in 2018:* Dr Sue Mann, 'Reproductive health: what women say', Public Health England, 28 June 2018, www.gov.uk/government/publications/reproductive-health-what-women-say.

36 *'Women are sexual slaves':* Shire Hite, *The Hite Report*, (Seven Stories Press, 1976).

CHAPTER 2: DON'T PUT UP WITH BAD SEX

43 *'I felt like I was being chewed on':* Lena Dunham, *Not That Kind of Girl* (HarperCollins, 2014), p. 55.

43 *Caitlin Moran refers to bad sex as 'the straight-up awful hump':* Caitlin Moran, 'Everything I know about sex', *Guardian*,

16 June 2018, www.theguardian.com/global/2018/jun/16/
caitlin-moran-everything-i-know-about-sex.

47 *forty-one per cent of videos (porn)':* Peggy Orenstein, *Girls &
Sex (Oneworld, 2016), pp. 34, 234.

51 *'When you slip on a banana peel':* Nora Ephron, *I Feel Bad
About My Neck: And Other Thoughts On Being a Woman*,
(Random House 2008).

53 Lyrics from 'Pull Up To My Bumper' by Grace Jones (Lyrics:
Grace Jones/ Kookoo Baya/Dana Manno).

54 Lyrics from 'Justify My Love' by Madonna (Lyrics: Ingrid
Chavez / Madonna).

55 Lyrics from 'Hounds of Love' by Kate Bush (Lyrics: Kate
Bush).

CHAPTER 3: HOW LIT IS YOUR CLIT?

61 *as Emma Watson says, 'it's worth it':* 'This is the sex education website that Emma Watson loves', *Marie Claire*, 23
July 2018, www.marieclaire.co.uk/news/omgyes-the-sex-
education-website-that-emma-watson-loves-15912.

62 *ten amazing facts about this nifty not-so-little organ:* Rachel
N. Pauls, 'Anatomy of the clitoris and the female sexual
response', *Clinical Anatomy*, 28(3) (2015), pp. 378–84.

68 *'I didn't begin enjoying sex':* 'Can you guess which celebrity spent $6,000 on sex toys?', *Marie Claire*, 23 October 2017,
www.marieclaire.co.uk/life/sex-and-relationships/celebrities-
sex-toys-546426.

72 *excitement levels were actually higher when using a sex toy:*
Carly Stern, 'Women orgasm 17% longer using a vibrator', *Mail
Online*, 30 September 2018, www.dailymail.co.uk/femail/
article-6224431/Women-orgasm-17-cent-LONGER-using-
vibrator.html.

CHAPTER 4: ORGASMS ARE A FEMINIST ISSUE

84   *'I'm a radical feminist, not the fun kind'*: Andrea Dworkin, 'Dworkin on Dworkin' from Radically Speaking: Feminism Reclaimed Ed. by Renate Klein and Diane Bell (Spinifex Press, 1996).

86   *'no woman gets an orgasm from shining the kitchen floor'*: Betty Friedan, The Feminine Mystique (W. W. Norton, 1963).

86   *So-called 'sex-positive' feminists of the Nineties:* Grace Banks, 'How Kathy Acker paved the way for women writing about their own experiences', The Pool, 21 September 2017, www.the-pool.com/arts-culture/books/2017/38/grace-banks-meets-chris-kraus-to-talk-kathy-acker; Susie Bright, Big Sex, Little Death (Seal Press, 2012).

86   *In The Female Eunuch Germaine Greer argues:* Germaine Greer, *The Female Eunuch* (Harper Collins, 1970).

87   *Susie Orbach's Fat Is a Feminist Issue skewered diet culture:* Susie Orbach, *Fat is A Feminist Issue* (Random House, 1978).

88   *Patricia Hill Collins wrote positively about motherhood:* Patricia Hill Collins, 'It's all in the family: intersections of gender, race, and nation', *Hypatia* 13(3) (1998), pp. 62–82.

88   *Gail Sheehy wrote prolifically about the menopause:* Gail Sheehy, *The Silent Passage: Menopause* (Random House, 1991).

88   *Caitlin Moran's book How to Be a Woman made feminist thinking funny*: Caitlin Moran, *How to Be a Woman* (Ebury, 2011).

89   *there are more men called John leading the UK's biggest companies:* Jennifer Rankin, 'Fewer women leading FTSE firms than men called John', *Guardian*, 6 March 2015, www.theguardian.com/business/2015/mar/06/johns-davids-and-ians-outnumber-female-chief-executives-in-ftse-100.

91 *the 'himpathy':* Kate Manne, 'Brett Kavanaugh and America's "himpathy" reckoning', *New York Times*, 26 September 2018, www.nytimes.com/2018/09/26/opinion/brett-kavanaugh-hearing-himpathy.html.

91 *'Because I am a woman':* Author Unknown, 'Clare Boothe Luce', Conneticut Women's Hall of Fame, Date Unknown. www.cwhf.org/inductees/politics-government-law/Clareboothe-luce#.XIT9LxP7TMI.

92 *'The system of patriarchy can function':* Gerda Lerner, *The Creation of Patriarchy* (Oxford University Press, 1987).

93 *Writer Naomi Wolf takes the argument a step further:* Naomi Wolf, *Vagina: A New Autobiography* (Virago, 2013).

CHAPTER 5: WHY SEX EDUCATION NEEDS TO GO BACK TO SCHOOL

103 *The British curriculum literally has not changed:* British Government, 'The national curriculum: other compulsory subjects', www.gov.uk/national-curriculum/other-compulsory-subjects.

103 *In 2016, British charity the Terrence Higgins Trust:* Terrence Higgins Trust, 'Relationships and sex education (RSE)', www.tht.org.uk/our-work/our-campaigns/relationships-and-sex-education-rse.

103 *Similarly, a report by the UK Youth Parliament:* UK Youth Parliament, *Are You Getting It?* (2007), www.ukyouthparliament.org.uk/wp-content/uploads/AreYouGettingIt.pdf.

104 *Thanks to a decision made in 2017:* Katherine Sellgren, 'Sex education to be compulsory in England's schools', BBC News, 1 March 2017, www.bbc.co.uk/news/education-39116783.

104 *an NSPCC report found that fifty-three per cent of young people:* Jack Hardy, 'Half of all children have watched porn online – including a quarter of 11-year-olds', *Independent*, 15

June 2016, www.independent.co.uk/news/uk/home-news/porn-children-pornography-online-nspcc-half-children-quarter-11-year-olds-a7082791.html.

105 *A huge UNESCO study of sex education courses:* UNESCO, *International Technical Guidance on Sexuality Education: An evidence-informed Approach for Schools, Teachers and Health Educators* (2009), unesdoc.unesco.org/images/0018/001832/183281e.pdf.

105 *'I'm not suggesting we teach children':* Jess Phillips MP, 'That Was Sh*t, Mate: With Jess Phillips MP', *The Hotbed* podcast, October 2018, www.itunes.apple.com/gb/podcast/that-was-s-t-mate-with-jess-phillips-mp/id1343455484?i=100042336994&mt=2.

107 *'This breaks my heart':* Brooke Seipel, 'Michelle Obama delivers message supporting girls education', *The Hill*, 23 September 2017.

108 *the lacy knickers worn by the complainant:* 'Irish outcry over teenager's underwear used in rape trial', BBC News, 14 November 2018, www.bbc.co.uk/news/world-europe-46207304.

108 *One journalist wrote about how she was asked to film a consent video:* Rachel King, 'Consent videos: why more and more men are asking women to record consent before sex', *London Evening Standard*, 22 October 2018 www.standard.co.uk/lifestyle/london-life/consent-videos-the-new-rules-of-engagement-a3968086.html.

109 *Tea Consent by Rockstar Dinosaur Pirate Princess:* Emmeline May, 'Consent: Not actually that complicated', Rockstar DinosaurPiratePrincess.com, 2 March 2015, www.rockstar dinosaurpirateprincess.com/2015/03/02/consent-not-actually-that-complicated.

113 *A connection has been found between the lack of adequate sex education:* Dr Eleanor Draeger, 'Getting relationships and sex education right for disabled young people', *National Chil-*

dren's Bureau, 8 January 2018, www.ncb.org.uk/news-opinion/news-highlights/getting-relationships-and-sex-education-right-disabled-young-people.

115 *'"Porn" is such a broad term'*: Alexander Bisley, 'Rashida Jones Interview: Hot Girls Wanted', 19 July 2017 www.vox. com/conversations/2017/7/19/15989210/rashida-jones-interview-hot-girls-wanted.

118 *The 'Reproduction' scene in Grease 2:* 'Grease 2 – reproduction scene', YouTube, uploaded 16 August 2016, www.youtube.com/watch?v=BwMoSPJ9Gjo.

CHAPTER 6: HOW SELF-IMAGE AFFECTS SEXY TIME

123 *'There is a gigantic difference'*: Jay Newton-Small, 'Palin's "good looking"', *Time*, 1 September 2008, www.swampland. time.com/2008/09/01/palins_good_looking.

123 *'Never mind Brexit, who won Legs-it?'*: Sarah Vine, 'One was relaxed, every inch a stateswoman while her opposite number was tense and uncomfortable: SARAH VINE says May v Sturgeon was a knockout victory for the PM', *Daily Mail*, 28 March 2017, www.dailymail.co.uk/debate/article-4354996/SARAH-VINE-says-v-Sturgeon-victory-PM.html.

123 *'Save the whales. Lose the blubber. Go vegetarian'*: Katherine Goldstein, 'PETA's new "Save the Whales" billboard takes aim at fat women', *Huffington Post*, 26 September 2009, www. huffingtonpost.co.uk/2009/08/26/petas-new-save-the-whales_n_261134.html?ec_carp=6486195083067389556.

124 *a recent study of bestselling children's stories:* Donna Ferguson, 'Must monsters always be male? Huge gender bias revealed in children's books', *Guardian*, 21 January 2018, www.theguardian.com/books/2018/jan/21/childrens-books-sexism-monster-in-your-kids-book-is-male.

125 *Girls with low body confidence:* Haroon Siddique, 'Poor body image makes girls less assertive and risks health, study finds', *Guardian*, 5 October 2017, www.theguardian.com/uk-news/2017/oct/05/poor-body-image-makes-girls-less-assertive-and-risks-health-study-finds.

127 *a 2008 study of nearly 2,000 adverts:* Julie M. Stankiewicz and Francine Rosselli, 'Women as sex objects and victims in print advertisements', *Sex Roles* 58(7–8) (2008), pp. 579–89.

127 *A 2017 study by J. Walter Thompson New York:* Katie Richards, 'Women continue to be sexualized and misrepresented in ads, even in 2017', *AdWeek*, 26 September 2017, www.adweek.com/brand-marketing/women-continue-to-be-sexualized-and-misrepresented-in-ads-even-in-2017.

128 *'The error that we tend to make':* Gloria Steinem, source unknown.

128 *some work by the YMCA:* Shivali Best, 'Around 60% of teens feel pressure to look "perfect" on social media – and influencers may be to blame', *Daily Mirror*, 23 July 2018, www.mirror.co.uk/tech/around-60-teens-feel-pressure-12965688.

128 *the Royal College of Psychiatrists are beginning to link:* Helen Chandler-Wilde, 'Regulate social media firms to protect young people's mental health, says Royal College of Psychiatrists', *Daily Telegraph*, 15 June 2018, www.telegraph.co.uk/news/2018/06/15/social-media-companies-must-regulated-stop-damaging-young-peoples.

128 *'Just because you are blind':* Margaret Cho, 'Beautiful,' MargaretCho.com 23 March 2006, www.margaretcho.com/2006/03/23/beautiful.

131 *One study describes body-image concerns:* Diana Sanchez and Amy Kiefer, 'Body concerns in and out of the bedroom: implications for sexual pleasure and problems', *Archives of Sexual Behavior* 36(6) (2007), pp. 808–20.

131 *Hang-ups about our body have been proven:* Chelsea D. Kiminik and Cindy M. Meston, 'Role of body esteem in the sexual excitation and inhibition responses of women with and without a history of childhood sexual abuse', *Journal of Sexual Medicine*, (13(11) (2016), 1718–28; William H. Masters and Virginia E. Johnson, *Human Sexual Inadequacy* (Little, Brown, 1970); Brooke Seal, Andrea Bradford and Cindy Meston, 'The association between body esteem and sexual desire among college women', *Archives of Sexual Behavior*, 38(5) (2009), pp. 866–72; Yasisca Pujols, Cindy M. Meston and Brooke N. Seal, 'The Association Between Sexual Satisfaction and Body Image in Women', *Journal of Sexual Medicine*, 7(2) (2010), pp. 905–16.

131 *Eating disorders among men:* 'Eating Disorders in Males', Eating Disorders website' www.eating-disorders.org.uk/ information/eating-disorders-in-males.

131 *calls to stop the 'short dick' jokes:* Dr Laurie Mintz, Becoming Cliterate (Harper Collins, 2017).

132 *Naomi Wolf clearly explains:* Naomi Wolf, Vagina: A New Autobiography (Virago, 2013).

133 *research by Harvard University lecturer Dr Justin Lehmiller:* Dr Justin Lehmiller, 'When do women orgasm during a hookup?', Lehmiller.com, 12 March 2014, www.lehmiller. com/blog/2014/3/5/when-do-women-orgasm-during-a-hookup-infographic.

135 *an actual swimsuit model's experience of sex:* Jenny Hare, *Orgasms and How to Have them: A Guide for Women* (Vision, 2007).

CHAPTER 7: THE SURPRISING POWER OF SEXUAL FANTASY

148 *A study by the University of Louvain in 2014:* Agata Blaszczak-Boxe, 'Sexy thoughts: the mind is key in female orgasm', *Live*

Science, 25 July 2014, www.livescience.com/47023-sexy-thoughts-mind-female-orgasm.html.

149 *a study in 2011 which surveyed 3,000 Australian female twins:* Brendan P. Zietsch, Geoffrey F. Miller, J. Michael Bailey and Nicholas G. Martin, 'Female orgasm rates are largely independent of other traits: implications for "female orgasmic disorder" and evolutionary theories of orgasm', *Journal of Sexual Medicine*, 8(8) (2011), pp. 2305–16.

149 *we strongly recommend that you read Nancy Friday's book:* Nancy Friday, *My Secret Garden: Women's Sexual Fantasies* (Pocket, 1978).

150 *A study in the Journal of Sexual Medicine:* Christian C. Joyal, Amélie Cossette and Vanessa Lapierre, 'What exactly is an unusual sexual fantasy?', *Journal of Sexual Medicine*, 12(2) (2015), pp. 328–40.

151 *including Women on Top in 1991:* Nancy Friday, *Women on Top* (Simon & Schuster, 1991).

152 *the book was banned from several libraries:* Herbert N. Foerstel, *Banned in the USA: A Reference Guide to Book Censorship in Schools and Public Libraries* (Greenwood Publishing Group, 2002).

152 *'In my sex fantasy':* Nora Ephron: *Crazy Salad: Some Things About Women,* (Knopf Publishing, 1975).

154 *355 college women at a north Texas university:* J. Bivona and J. Critelli, 'The nature of women's rape fantasies: an analysis of prevalence, frequency, and contents', *Journal of Sexual Research*, 46(1) (2009), pp. 33–45.

CHAPTER 8: CUNNILINGUS: TRICKY WORD, EASY ORGASM

161 *oral sex is one of the reasons attributed:* Hannah Jane Parkinson, 'Do lesbians have better sex than straight women?',

Guardian, 9 July 2018, www.theguardian.com/lifeandstyle/ 2018/jul/09/do-lesbians-have-better-sex-than-straight-women; Eleanor Margolis, 'Five theories as to why lesbians are more likely to orgasm than straight women', *New Statesman*, 21 August 2014, www.newstatesman.com/scitech/2014/08/five-theories-why-lesbians-are-more-likely-orgasm-straight-women.

164 *In 2016 researchers Ruth Lewis and Cicely Martin conducted:* Ruth Lewis and Cicely Martin, 'Oral sex, young people and gendered narratives of reciprocity', *Journal of Sex Research*, 53(7) (2016), pp. 776–87.

166 *It doesn't help that Sigmund Freud:* Sigmund Freud, *Three Essays on the Theory of Sexuality*, 1905.

169 Lyrics from 'Work It' by Missy Elliot/Timbaland (Lyrics: Missy Elliot).

169 Lyrics from 'Twist' by Goldfrapp (Lyrics: Alison Goldfrapp).

169 Lyrics from 'Taste' by Bikini Kill (Lyrics: Kathleen Hanna).

169 Lyrics from 'Not Tonight' by L'il Kim (Songwriting: K. Jones, M. Elliott, L. Lopes, S. Harris, A. Martinez, R. Bell, G. Brown, M. Muhammed, C. Smith, J. Taylor, D. Thomas, E. Toon).

CHAPTER 9: EVERYTHING YOU WANT TO KNOW ABOUT BUM SEX BUT WERE TOO BRITISH TO ASK

178 *anal sex is riskier than other forms of shagging:* 'Does anal sex have any health risks?', NHS website, www.nhs.uk/common-health-questions/sexual-health/does-anal-sex-have-any-health-risks.

179 Lyrics from 'Anaconda' by Nicki Minaj (Lyrics: O. Maraj, J. Jones, J. Solone-Myvett, E.Clark, M. Palacios, A. Ray).

180 *Anal action is on the rise for straight men:* K. R. McBride and J. D. Fortenberry, 'Heterosexual anal sexuality and anal sex behaviors: a review', *Journal of Sexual Research*, 47(2) (2010), pp. 123–36.

181 *Andrea Dworkin famously wrote:* Andrea Dworkin, *Intercourse* (Free Press, 1987).

184 *In the 2017 study of heterosexual women's views:* Kimberley R. MacBride, 'Heterosexual women's anal sex attitudes and motivations: a focus group study', *Journal of Sex Research* (August 2017), pp.1–11.

185 *an increased risk of infection after douching:* H. Hambrick et al., 'Rectal douching among men who have sex with men in Paris: implications for HIV/STI risk behaviors and rectal microbicide development', *AIDS and Behavior*, 22(2) (2017), pp. 379–87.

186 *Finally, an extra top tip:* 'I'd Like Something Up My Bottom, Please', *The Hotbed* podcast, 21 March 2018, www.itunes. apple.com/gb/podcast/id-like-something-up-my-bottom-please/id1343455484?i=1000407010122&mt=2.

CHAPTER 10: PORN: FEELS SO RIGHT, SEEMS SO WRONG

192 *'I think porn, like anything else':* Emily Hewett 'Scarlett Johansson: Women can enjoy porn too'. *Metro*, 7 November 2013. www.metro.co.uk/2013/11/07/scarlett-johansson-women-can-enjoy-porn-too-4177202.

192 *We did an episode: The Hotbed* podcast, Can Feminist Porn Give You The Horn?, 14 March 2018 www.itunes.apple.com/gb/podcast/can-feminist-porn-give-you-the-horn/id1343455484?i=1000406304438&mt=2.

194 *As data journalist Mona Chalabi says:* Mona Chalabi and Mae Ryan, 'The Vagina Dispatches', *Guardian*, 2016, www.the-guardian.com/lifeandstyle/series/vagina-dispatches.

195 *One study used eye-movement trackers:* Akira Tsujimura et al., 'Sex differences in visual attention to sexually explicit videos: a preliminary study', *Journal of Sexual Medicine*, 6(4) (2009), pp. 1011–17.

195 *In another study, men and women were asked:* Heather Rupp and Kim Wallen, 'Sex differences in response to visual sexual stimuli: a review', *Archives of Sexual Behavior*, 37(2) (2007), pp. 206–18.

196 *refers to 'F**kability v Invisibility':* Gail Dines, 'Growing Up in a Pornified Culture', TEDxNavesink, YouTube, 28 April 2015.

196 *could be the reason why labiaplasty:* Ozan Dogan and Murat Yassa, 'Major motivators and sociodemographic features of women undergoing labiaplasty', *Aesthetic Surgery Journal* (December 2018); Weck Turini et al., 'The impact of labiaplasty on sexuality', Plastic and Reconstructive Surgery, 141(1) (2018), pp. 592e-3e.

197 *some studies suggest that many people:* Luke Sniewski, Panteá Farvid and Phil Carter, 'The assessment and treatment of adult heterosexual men with self-perceived problematic pornography use: a review', *Addictive Behaviors*, 77 (2018), pp. 217–24; Harold Rosenberg and Shane Kraus, 'The relationship of "passionate attachment" for pornography with sexual compulsivity, frequency of use, and craving for pornography', *Addictive Behaviors*, 39(5) (2014), pp. 1012–17; Marie-Pier Vaillancourt-Morel and Sophie Bergeron, 'Self-perceived problematic pornography use: beyond individual differences and religiosity', *Archives of Sexual Behavior*, 48(2) (2019), pp.437–41.

198 *'Since the advent of the internet':* Paula Hall, 'We Need To Talk About Porn Addiction', TEDxLeamington Spa, YouTube, 29 March 2016, www.youtube.com/watch?v=-Qf2e3XZ-8Tw.

198 An academic study in 2018: Eran Shor and Golshan Golriz, 'Gender, race and aggression in mainstream pornography', *Archives of Sexual Behavior* (September 2018).

199 *A 2011 study of nearly 3,000 American men:* Neil Malamuth, Gert Hald and Mary Koss, 'Pornography, individual differences in risk and men's acceptance of violence against women in a representative sample', *Sex Roles*, 66(8) (2011), pp.427–39.

199 *Naomi Wolf writes about this:* Naomi Wolf, Vagina: A New Autobiography (Virago, 2013).

206 *Jon Ronson's 'The Butterfly Effect':* Jon Ronson, The Butterfly Effect podcast, 2017, www.itunes.apple.com/gb/podcast/the-butterfly-effect-with-jon-ronson/id1258779354?mt=2; Gail Dines, Pornland: How Porn Hijacked Our Sexuality (Beacon Press, 2011).

207 *The International Union of Sex Workers campaigns:* 'Our Aim', The International Union of Sex Workers website, 17 December 2014 www.iusw.org.

207 *a survey by the NSPCC found:* Katherine Sellgren, 'Pornography "desensitising" young people', BBC News, 15 June 2016, www.bbc.co.uk/news/education-36527681.

208 *Pornhub reported that thirty-seven per cent:* '2018 year in review', Pornhub, 11 December 2018, www.pornhub.com/insights/2018-year-in-review.

209 *a conversation between pornographer and artist:* Annie Sprinkle, 'My conversation with an anti-porn feminist', www.anniesprinkle.org/my-conversation-with-an-anti-porn-feminist.

210 *'Guy: So ... what do you do for fun?':* @MichaelaCoel on Twitter.

CHAPTER 11: COMING TOGETHER AND OTHER LIES

218 *A 2018 survey by the University of California:* University of California, *Hollywood Diversity Report 2018*, www.socialsciences.ucla.edu/wp-content/uploads/2018/02/UC-LA-Hollywood-Diversity-Report-2018-2-27-18.pdf.

219 *when it was said during an episode:* Stephen LaConte, 'Crazy Ex-Girlfriend just made television history by saying the word "clitoris"', *Buzzfeed*, 22 October 2017, www.buzzfeed.com/stephenlaconte/rachel-bloom-from-crazy-ex-girlfriend-had-to-fight-the-cw.

219 *It shouldn't be noteworthy:* Benjamin Lee, 'Viola Davis: I stifled who I was for years to be seen as pretty. I lost years', *Guardian*, 20 October 2018, www.theguardian.com/film/2018/oct/20/viola-davis-stifled-who-was-lost-years-the-help.

219 *It was coined by Laura Mulvey in 1975:* Laura Mulvey, 'Visual pleasure and narrative cinema', *Screen*, 16(3) (October 1975).

220 *'It's a struggle every day':* Tara Aquino, 'Jill Soloway's Honest Look at Female Sexuality, "Afternoon Delight," Is a Sign of Things to Come' , Complex.com, 10 September 2013.

221 *A survey of 4,400 people:* Susanna Weiss, *How Achievable is Simultaneous Orgasm, Really?* Glamour, 21 March 2017, www.glamour.com/story/how-achievable-is-simultaneous-orgasm.

221 *ten per cent of women:* Stuart Brody and Petr Weiss, 'Simultaneous penile—vaginal orgasm is associated with sexual satisfaction', *Journal of Sexual Medicine*, 9(9) (2012), pp. 734—41.

223 *A good example of the limits:* M. Asher Cantrell, '10 famous films that surprisingly fail the bechdel test', Film School Rejects, www.filmschoolrejects.com/10-famous-films-that-surprisingly-fail-the-bechdel-test-e54ceo02bcfc.

CHAPTER 12: SNOGGING: WE NEED IT, WE WANT IT

230 *Statistics from a survey of 27,000 people:* Gisele Galoustian, 'Think millennials are the hookup generation?', University of Florida, 8 February 2016, www.fau.edu/newsdesk/articles/millennials-sex-study.php.

233 *'I am a strong believer in kissing':* Claudya Martinez, 11 Jennifer Lopez Quotes About Life, Love and Parenting, *Mom.Me*, 19 November 2015. www.mom.me/entertainment/25161-jennifer-lopez-quotes-life-love-parenting/item/jennifer-lopez-quotes-dating.

234 *it offers a raft of benefits:* Adrienne Santos-Longhurst, '16 reasons to smooch: how kissing benefits your health', *Healthline*, 10 July 2018, www.healthline.com/health/benefits-of-kissing.

CHAPTER 13: I BLAME THE HORMONES

242 *Oxytocin is known as 'the love hormone':* 'Hormones in labour', NCT website, www.nct.org.uk/labour-birth/your-guide-labour/hormones-labour.

243 *Hormones are naturally occurring chemicals:* 'Hormones in human reproduction', BBC website, www.bbc.com/bitesize/guides/zs9hb82/revision/1.

244 *some studies have found that testosterone levels:* Menelaos L. Batrinos, 'Testosterone and aggressive behavior in man', International Journal of Endocrinology and Metabolism, 10(3) (2012), pp. 563–8.

244 *Loss of sex drive in men:* 'Loss of libido', NHS website, www.nhs.uk/conditions/loss-of-libido/.

244 *Many trans women find:* Mats Holmberg, Stefan Arver and Cecilia Dhejne, 'Supporting sexuality and improving sexual function in transgender persons', *Nature Reviews Urology*, 16(2) (2019), pp. 121–39.

245 *the oxytocin released in your body:* 'Sex chemistry "lasts two years"', BBC News, 1 February 2006, www.news.bbc.co.uk/1/hi/4669104.stm.

245 *As women go through menopause:* 'Menopause', NHS website, www.nhs.uk/conditions/menopause.

246 *'The problem with looking in the mirror':* Chimamanda Ngozi Adichie, 'What I see in the mirror', *Guardian*, 23 January 2010, www.theguardian.com/lifeandstyle/2010/jan/23/chimamanda-ngozi-adichie-interview.

247 Follicle-stimulating hormone (FSH) and luteinising hormone (LH): 'What happens to girls and boys', NHS website, www.nhs.uk/live-well/sexual-health/stages-of-puberty-what-happens-to-boys-and-girls/; 'Puberty for girls', Childline website, www.childline.org.uk/info-advice/you-your-body/puberty/puberty-girls.

249 *Taking the combined pill:* 'Combined contraceptive pill', NHS website, www.nhs.uk/conditions/contraception/combined-contraceptive-pill.

253 *As you approach menopause:* 'Menopause', NHS website, www.nhs.uk/conditions/menopause/treatment.

CHAPTER 14: THE PELVIC FLOOR: BEAR WITH US

259 *Look after your pelvic floor muscles:* Yanlei Ma and Huanlong Qin, 'Pelvic floor muscle exercises may improve female sexual function', *Medical Hypotheses*, 72(2) (2009), p. 223.

263 *It is also thought that a strong pelvic floor:* 'Pelvic floor exercises', Tommy's charity website, date unknon, www.tommys.org/pregnancy-information/im-pregnant/exercise-pregnancy/pelvic-floor-exercises.

264 *severe pelvic floor dysfunction:* 'Pelvic organ prolapse', NHS website, www.nhs.uk/conditions/pelvic-organ-prolapse.

265 *Any bit of accidental weeing:* Elizabeth Davies, 'What is the pelvic floor and why does it matter?', The Hotbed Collective website, 1 March 2018, www.thehotbedcollective.com/single-post/2018/03/01/What-Is-The-Pelvic-Floor-and-Why-Does-It-Matter.

CHAPTER 15: LONG-TERM LOVERS: THE REALITY

280 *'People have known love forever':* Miranda Sawyer, 'Esther Perel: "Fix the sex and your relationship will transform"', Guardian, 30 September 2018, www.theguardian.com/life-andstyle/2018/sep/30/esther-perel-fix-the-sex-and-your-relationship-will-transform-esther-perel.

281 *One of the most googled phrases:* 'Can a sexless marriage survive?', *Irish Independent*, 22 August 2018.

283 *Basson argues that sexual response:* Sarah Barmak, 'The misunderstood science of sexual desire', *The Cut*, 26 April 2018, www.thecut.com/2018/04/the-misunderstood-science-of-sexual-desire.html.

284 *the importance of the 'maintenance shag':* 'The Maintenance Shag: With Sali Hughes', *The Hotbed* podcast, 21 November 2018, www.itunes.apple.com/gb/podcast/the-maintenance-shag-with-sali-hughes/id1343455484?i=1000424270272&mt=2.

285 *'The very thought of you has my legs spread':* Rupi Kaur, *Milk and Honey* (Andrews McMeel Publishing, 2015).

286 *'When the impulse to share becomes obligatory':* Esther Perel, *Mating in Captivity: How to Keep Desire and Passion Alive in Long-Term Relationships* (Hodder & Stoughton, 2007).

287 *'Sexual currency is the things you'd only do':* 'Dr Karen, Dr Karen, Dr Karen', The Hotbed podcast, 8 August 2018, www.itunes.apple.com/gb/podcast/dr-karen-dr-karen-dr-karen/id1343455484?i=1000417401042&mt=2.

CHAPTER 16: GROWING OLD DISGRACEFULLY

298 *there's a 'golden ratio':* Pamela M. Pallett, Stephen Link and Kang Lee, 'New "golden" ratios for facial beauty', *Vision Research*, 50(2) (2010), p. 149.

299 *'I feel exactly like I've always felt, except better':* India Knight, *In Your Prime: Older, Happier, Wiser* (Penguin, 2014).

300 *Whoopi Goldberg, actress and presenter of The View:* Whoopi Goldberg, *If Someone Says 'You Complete Me': Run!: Whoopi's Big Book of Relationships* (Hachette, 2015).

301 *'Life's too fucking short to get depressed':* Janet Street-Porter, *Life's Too F***ing Short* (Quadrille, 2009).

302 *'First of all, we're braver':* Jill Lawless, 'Jane Fonda says sex improves with age: "We're braver — what the heck do we have to lose?"', *Toronto Sun*, 1 September 2017.

303 *'We'll probably be livid with ourselves':* Sophie Heawood, 'What I'll be doing differently in 2016, *The Pool*, 2 January 2016.

306 *An American study found that half:* Stacy Tessler Lindau et al., 'A study of sexuality and health among older adults in the United States', *New England Journal of Medicine*, 357 (2007), pp. 762–74.

307 *'All this stuff is made doubly, triply confusing':* Miranda Sawyer, *Out of Time: Midlife, If You Still Think You're Young* (Fourth Estate, 2016).

308 *any benefits of this are outweighted by horrible side effects:* Stephen Levine, 'Flibanserin', *Archives of Sexual Behavior*, 44(8) (2015), pp. 2107–9; Holly L. Thacker, Adriane Fugh-Berman and Alessandra Hirsch, 'Should ob/gyns prescribe flibanserin for their patients?', *Contemporary OB/GYN*, 61(8) (August 2016).

308 *'At seventy-four, I have never had such a fulfilling sex life':* Author Unknown, 'Jane Fonda's Rampant Sex Life at 74',

The Sun, 10 July 2012 www.thesun.co.uk/sol/homepage/
showbiz/4420885/Jane-Fondas-rampant-sex-life-at-74.
html.

308 *One study, which tracked 800 women:* Rick Nauert, 'Sexual
satisfaction in older women: it's complicated', *Psych Central*,
www.psychcentral.com/news/2012/01/04/sexual-satisfac-
tion-in-older-women-its-complicated/33267.html.

CHAPTER 17: THE FUTURE OF SEX:
WHERE DO WE GO FROM HERE?

316 *'Another world is not only possible':* Arundhati Roy, *An
Ordinary Person's Guide to Empire* (Flamingo, 2004).

317 *'They [the dolls] don't possess any of the unpleasant qualities':* Julie Beck, 'Married to a doll: why one man advocates
synthetic love', *The Atlantic*, September 2013, www.theat-
lantic.com/health/archive/2013/09/married-to-a-doll-why-
one-man-advocates-synthetic-love/279361.

319 *Alys outlines why technology isn't the thing:* 'Why You
Should Be Excited About the Future of Sex', *TEDx Covent
GardenWomen*, YouTube, 9 March 2018, www.youtube.
com/watch?v=A40JbaaM4ZE.

320 *It hit the headlines when it won a prize:* Jen Copesake, 'CES
2019: "Award-winning" sex toy for women withdrawn from
show', BBC News, 9 January 2019, www.bbc.co.uk/news/
technology-46809807.

RESOURCES

Here you will find links to sources for information, charities and further reading/podcasts on a number of topics.

PELVIC FLOOR

Pelvic Obstetric and Gynaecological Physiotherapy
www.pogp.csp.org.uk

This is a register of all qualified women's health physiotherapists in Great Britain, and also where you can find information on pelvic floor dysfunction and physio moves you can try at home.

NHS website
www.nhs.uk/conditions/pelvic-organ-prolapse

The NHS website has lots of information about pelvic floor health and dysfunction.

'What's the Pelvic Floor and Why Does It Matter?'
www.thehotbedcollective.com/single-post/2018/03/01/
What-Is-The-Pelvic-Floor-and-Why-Does-It-Matter

An article on our website which details symptoms of pelvic floor dysfunction

The Pelvic Floor Bible by Jane Simpson

This book, published in 2019 by Penguin, is a guide to pelvic floor health by continence specialist Jane Simpson.

'The Pelvic Paw Patrol'
www.itunes.apple.com/gb/podcast/pelvic-paw-patrol-how-to-get-in-mood-pelvic-floor-health/id1343455484?i=10004
4125244&mt=2

This is an episode of our podcast, *The Hotbed*, in which we speak to women's health and fitness expert Dr Amal Hassan and post-natal personal trainer Elizabeth Davies about the pelvic floor.

SEXUAL ABUSE/TRAUMA

If you are in immediate danger, please call 999 to speak to the police. If you feel you might harm yourself, please call 116 123 to speak to the Samaritans.

Rape Crisis England and Wales
www.rapecrisis.org.uk
Helpline: 0808 802 9999

A national helpline for women and girls who have experienced rape or sexual assault. Phone them or check their website for face-to-face support closest to you.

The National Male Survivor Helpline by Safeline
www.safeline.org.uk
Helpline: 0808 800 5005

Telephone support for male survivors of rape or sexual abuse.

The Young People's Helpline by Safeline
www.safeline.org.uk
Helpline: 0808 800 5007

Telephone for young survivors of rape or sexual abuse.

Havoca
havoca.org

Online resources for adult victims of child sexual abuse.

The Survivors' Trust
thesurvivorstrust.org

A UK-wide national umbrella agency for 130 specialist organisations which support the impact of rape, sexual violence and childhood sexual abuse throughout the UK and Ireland.

Galop
www.galop.org.uk
Helpline: 0800 999 5428

Charity supporting LGBTQIA+ victims of sexual and domestic violence.

100 Women I Know
www.100womeniknow.com

A website, film and book giving voice to female victims of rape and sexual abuse. Proceeds from book sales (publisher: Break the Habit Press) go towards funding consent workshops for young people.

SH! Women's Store
www.sh-womenstore.com/blog/advice

This London-based sex shop holds workshops on sex skills as well as on building up body and sexual confidence after sexual abuse.

SEX AND RELATIONSHIPS

If you feel you need therapy around sex and/or relationships, and if you feel comfortable to do so, you can speak to your doctor in the first instance. They can advise on physical issues and refer you to 'talking therapy' for an issue such as anxiety or depression. You may even be able to get a referral for sex therapy, although it depends on which area you live in whether you can get one on the NHS or not.

NHS
www.nhs.uk/common-health-questions/sexual-health/what-does-a-sex-therapist-do

NHS information about what sex therapy can do.

College of Sexual and Relationship Therapists
www.cosrt.org.uk

Directory of sex and relationship therapists in the UK.

Relate
www.relate.org.uk

Sex and relationships charity providing affordable face-to-face and online or telephone counselling, and sex therapy.

The British Association of Counselling and Psychotherapy
www.bacp.co.uk

An online directory of all therapists and counsellors who are members of this body, listed by area, price and specialisation.

The Havelock Clinic
thehavelockclinic.com
Information: 0207 467 8354

Private clinic run by Dr Karen Gurney, the Hotbed Collective's resident psychotherapist and psychosexologist, and her team of doctors, psychosexual counsellors and psychologists doing sex therapy. Their services are available face-to-face in London, online or via Skype.

The Hotbed podcast
www.itunes.apple.com/gb/podcast/the-hotbed

This is our podcast which regularly features experts in the field of sex and relationships as well as first-hand stories and some silliness.

Where Should We Begin? podcast
www.estherperel.com/podcast

We also love Esther Perel's podcast, which is recorded in real therapy sessions with her clients.

Unexpected Fluids podcast
www.bbc.co.uk/programmes/p066mgz9

Our friend Alix Fox has a brilliant podcast about when sex goes awry.

Salty magazine
www.saltyworld.net

We love this online magazine about sexuality in all its shapes and forms.

CONTRACEPTION AND SEXUALLY TRANSMITTED INFECTIONS

The Family Planning Association
www.fpa.org.uk

Information on sex education, birth control and reproductive rights.

Brook
www.brook.org.uk

Sex advice for people under twenty-five.

Terrence Higgins Trust
www.tht.org.uk

Information and online counselling for people living with HIV.

British Association of Sexual Health and HIV
www.bashh.org

Information on good sexual health.

GUM Clinic directory
www.nhs.uk/service-search/sexual-health-informa-
tion-and-support/locationsearch/734

NHS search engine for finding a sexual health clinic near you.

FEMALE GENITAL MUTILATION

NHS
www.nhs.uk/conditions/female-genital-mutilation-fgm

NHS factsheet about FGM.

Daughters of Eve
www.dofeve.org

Charity raising awareness and signposting support for victims
of FGM.

Forward UK
www.forwarduk.org.uk/key-issues/fgm

African-led women's rights organisation with FGM as one of its
priority issues.

PORN

The Porn Conversation
www.thepornconversation.org

Website set up by feminist porn-maker Erika Lust with information and age-appropriate suggestions of how to talk to kids and young people about porn.

Bish
www.bishuk.com

Website with clear information and video guides for young people on topics such as porn, safe sex and anatomy.

GENDER AND SEXUALITY

LGBT Foundation
www.lgbt.foundation

National charity providing support and information for the lesbian, gay, bisexual and trans community.

Stonewall
www.stonewall.org.uk

Information, training and lobbying organisation for lesbian, gay, bisexual and trans rights.

TransUnite
www.transunite.co.uk

Directory of trans support groups across the UK.

VAGINISMUS

NHS
www.nhs.uk/conditions/vaginismus

NHS factsheet about vaginismus, including when to get help and what will happen at the doctor's appointment.

Vaginismus Awareness`
www.vaginismusawareness.com

Charity providing information and support to those with vaginismus.

ANORGASMIA

NHS
www.nhs.uk/common-health-questions/sexual-health/what-can-cause-orgasm-problems-in-women

NHS factsheet about orgasm problems in women, possible causes and when to get help.

BODY IMAGE

NHS
www.nhs.uk/conditions/body-dysmorphia

NHS factsheet about body dysmorphia.

Mind
www.mind.org.uk

Mental health charity with information and support for a wide range of mental health problems, including those related to eating disorders and/or body image.

Beat
www.beateatingdisorders.org.uk
Charity supporting those with eating disorders.

Just Eat It: How Intuitive Eating Can Help You Get Your Shit Together Around Food by Laura Thomas, PhD
Great book, published by Bluebird, which helps to skewer diet culture and foster a healthy attitude around food.

Some body-positive Instagram accounts to follow:

@theslumflower

@bodyposipanda

@getyourskinout

@scarrednotscared

CONSENT

Rockstar Dinosaur Pirate Princess
'Tea Consent' video www.youtube.com/watch?time_continue=6&v=fGoWLWS4-kU
Animated video of the Tea Consent blog we published in the sex education chapter.

ACKNOWLEDGEMENTS

ANNIKI AND LISA THANK:

Cherry Healey, for getting us together and for being our loudest, most passionate and cheekiest cheerleader. Dr Karen Gurney, for taking on three massive idiots and for being so generous with your time, wisdom and cocktail-making. Rowan Yapp, for finding us and for helping us write a book we are so proud of. Chloe, Harriet, Anna and the rest of the Penguin gang, you are wonderful and we couldn't have done it without you (sorry about all the Michael Hutchence references). Vic, for the beautiful illustrations and for sending us an email containing the words 'hand-drawn bum hole'. Anna at Ultra Violet, for sharing the mental load of the Hotbed podcast. Alex Graham and Shola Aleje = the world's best podcast producers. Wingwoman Elizabeth Adetula. Sophie and Ayoub at Acast.

Our wonderful Instagram followers and podcast listeners for your support and your honesty. Nancy Friday for the inspiration.

ANNIKI THANKS:

Paul (for putting up with me sharing our stories), Rae and Greta, my lovely daughters, Mum (who won't read any of this I hope), Dad, John, Marylyn, my sisters Camille, Sophie, Katherine, all my friends and family and Lisa who has been the perfect 'work wife', and continues to be a joy to work with.

LISA THANKS:

My three best boys. Mum and Mark. Sarah. My dad and my father-in-law: I miss you. My mother-in-law, my aunties and everyone who helps look after me and my family. Anniki: the Howard to my Gary, thank you for reminding me that the brief was 'uplifting'. Mum: as long as you like this book, I'll be happy.

penguin.co.uk/vintage